Adu[illegible] Children of Toxic Parents

How to Establish Boundaries, Reclaim Your Emotional Autonomy, and Heal from Distant, Rejecting, Emotionally Immature Parents.

Jacqueline D. Austin

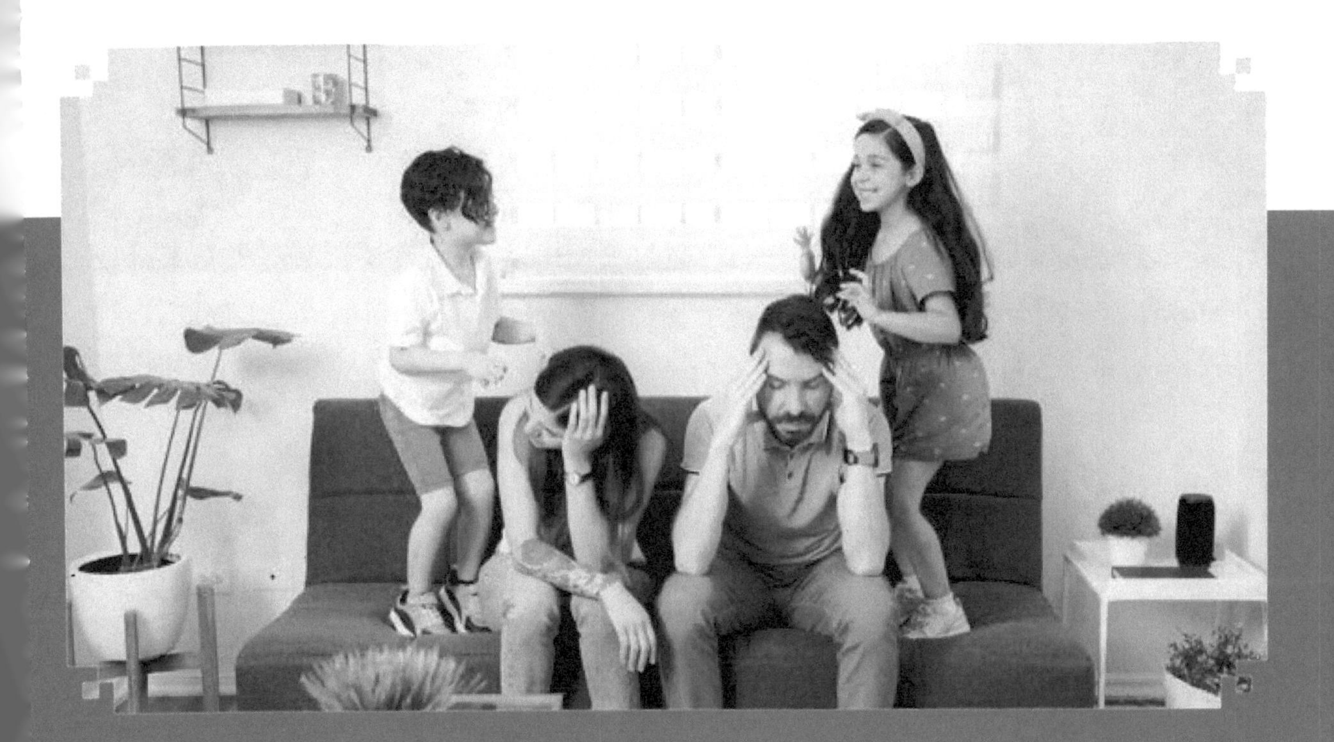

Manufactured in: USA

Interior Design: DANIELLE REES

Cover Art: DANIELLE REES

Art Producer: BROOKE WHITE

Production Editor: SIENNA ADAMS

Editor: AALIYAH LYONS

Production Manager: SARAH JOHNSON

Photography: MICHAEL SMITH

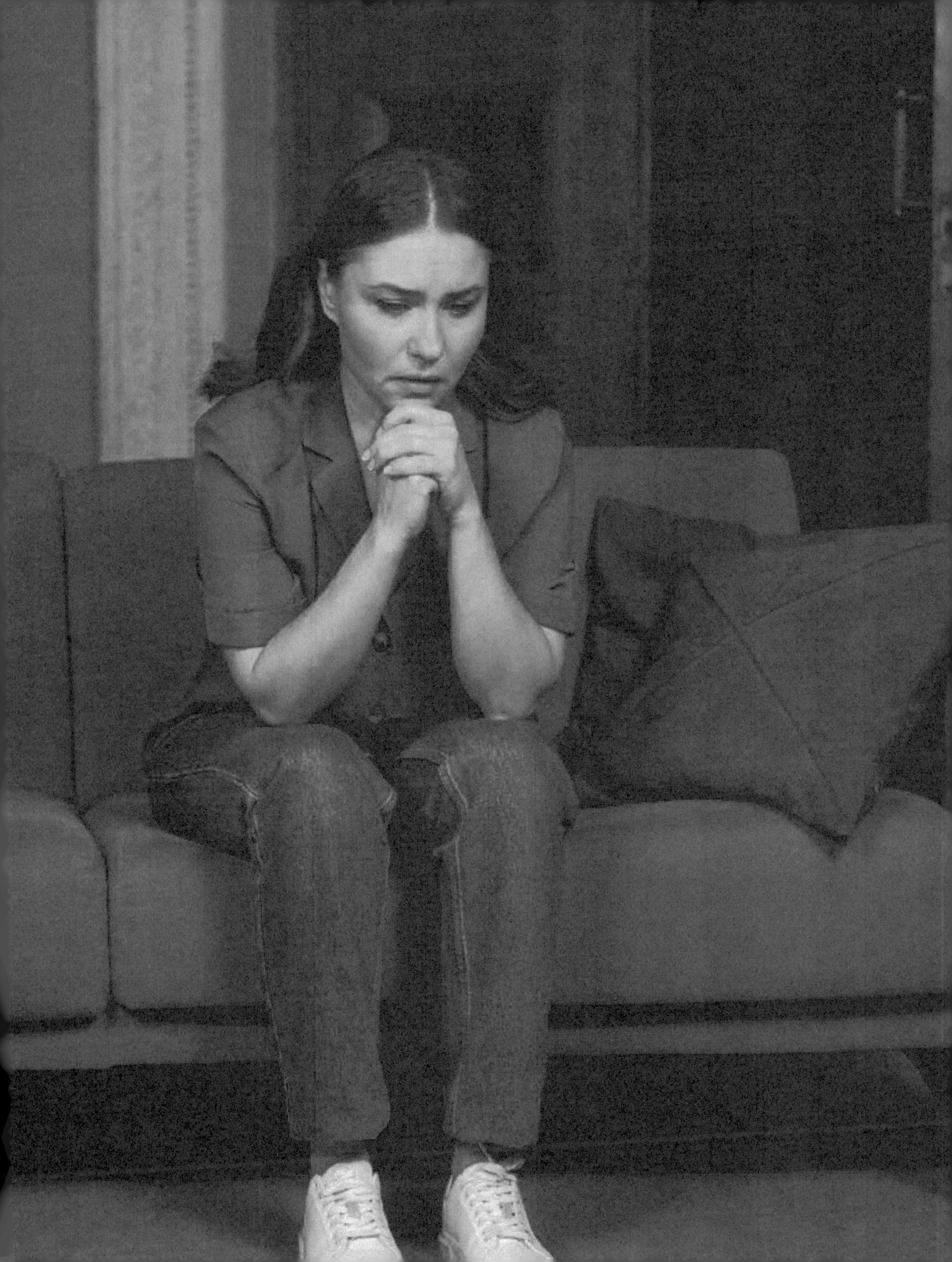

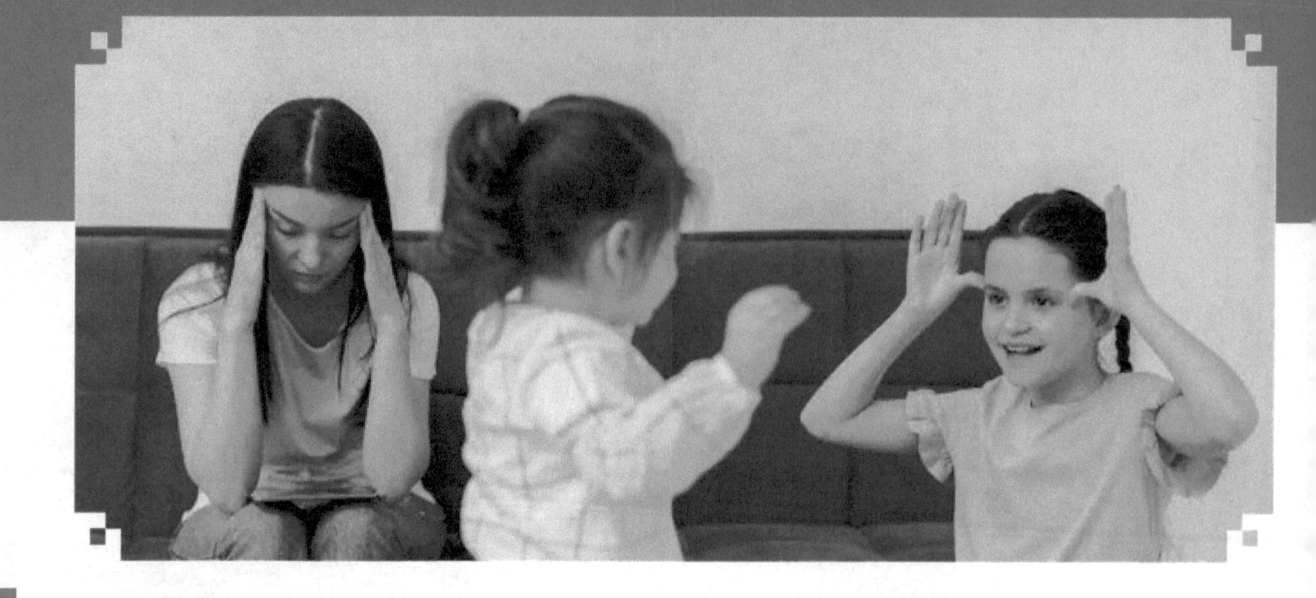

Table Of Contents

Introduction 1

Chapter 1
Understanding Toxic Parenting 3
What Makes a Parent Toxic? 4
Common Traits of Toxic Parents 5
The Psychological and Emotional Impact on Adult Children 7
Understanding the Impact of Toxic Parenting 8
Real-life Stories: Recognizing Toxic Behavior in Parents 9

Chapter 2
Types of Toxic Parents 11
The Narcissistic Parent 12
Coping Strategies 12
The Controlling Parent 13
Actions to Take to Get One's Freedom Back 13
The Emotionally Immature Parent 13
The Abusive Parent 14
The Distant or Rejecting Parent 15

Chapter 3
Recognizing the Effects on Your Life 16
Identifying Toxic Patterns in Your Behavior 18
The Impact on Self-Esteem and Self-Worth 20
Relationship Challenges Stemming from Toxic Parenting 21
Breaking the Cycle: Avoiding Toxic Patterns in Your Own Parenting 23

Chapter 4
Establishing Boundaries 26
The Importance of Setting Boundaries 27

How to Establish and Maintain Healthy Boundaries 28
Dealing with Resistance and Guilt 29
Practical Exercises for Boundary Setting 31
Case Studies: Success Stories in Boundary Setting 33

Chapter 5
Reclaiming Your Emotional Autonomy 37
Understanding Emotional Autonomy 38
Steps to Reclaiming Your Emotional Independence 38
Techniques for Self-Validation and Self-Care 40
Building Emotional Intelligence 42
Mindfulness Practices for Emotional Health 44

Chapter 6
Healing from the Past 46
The Journey of Healing 47
Working Through Feelings of Anger and Resentment 48
Forgiveness: What It Is and What It Isn't 49
Seeking Professional Help and Support 50
Therapeutic Techniques: CBT, EMDR, and More 51

Chapter 7
Overcoming Guilt and Shame 53
Understanding the Origins of Guilt and Shame 54
Differentiating Between Healthy and Unhealthy Guilt 55
Strategies for Letting Go of Shame 56
Rebuilding a Positive Self-Image 58
Seeking Support and Sharing Your Story 62

Chapter 8
Building Resilience and Inner Strength 64
Developing a Resilient Mindset 65
Coping Strategies for Difficult Times 67
The Role of Self-Compassion in Building Strength 68
Finding Meaning and Purpose After Trauma 70
Techniques for Sustaining Long-Term Resilience 72

Chapter 9
Building Healthy Relationships 73
Forming New, Healthy Relationship Patterns 74
The Role of Communication in Healthy Relationships 74
Finding and Nurturing Supportive Friendships 74
Identifying and Avoiding Toxic Relationships 75
Building Trust and Intimacy 75

Chapter 10
Moving Forward 76
Embracing Your New Life 77
Setting Goals for Personal Growth and Fulfillment 77
Celebrating Your Progress and Successes 77
Developing a Positive Mindset 77
Long-term Strategies for Maintaining Emotional Health 77

Chapter 11
Resources for Further Support 78
Recommended Books 79
Online Support Groups 79
Online Resources and Communities 79
Apps and Tools for Emotional Health 80
Building Your Support Network 80
Conclusion 81

Introduction

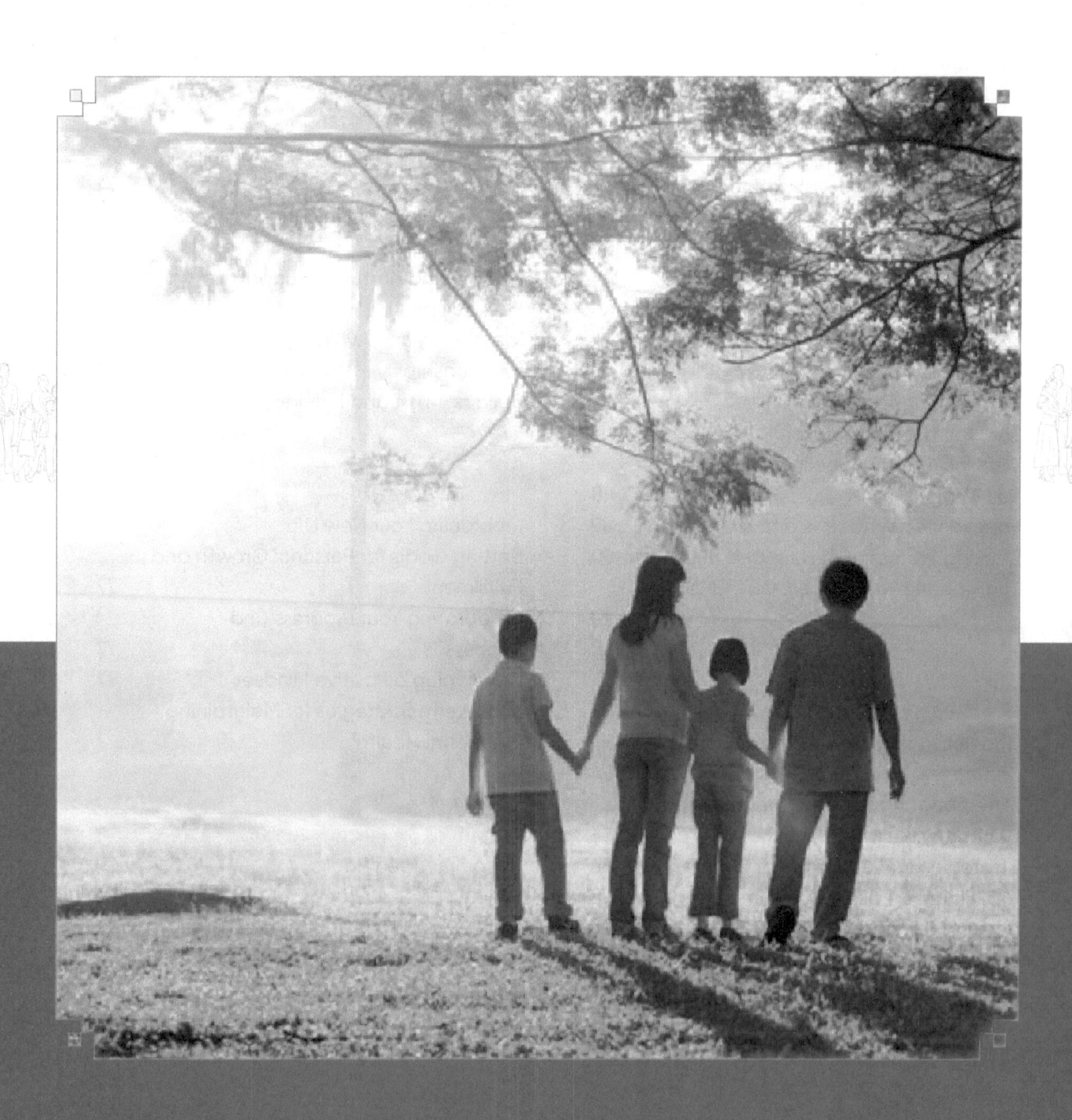

Living as an adult is already challenging, and it can be more difficult with unresolved emotional wounds from childhood. For people who grew up with toxic parents, meaning distant, rejecting, and emotionally immature parents, adulthood can be challenging. The effects of poisonous parenting can cause deep scars, shaping someone's self-perception and overall life. Toxic parents behave in ways that cause guilt, fear or obligation in their children. This parenting pattern full of fear, shame and emotional neglect is called poisonous parenting.

The biggest problem of growing up with toxic parents is that it can create lifelong effects that control the ways we experience our adulthoods, even if we are unaware of it. Parents who might be distant, rejecting or emotionally immature are likely to do emotions that focus on love and acceptance and leave their children unworthy and confused. If you are an adult child of toxic parents, then don't be too surprised if you are paralyzed by self-doubt, cannot set proper boundaries, and crave a sense of emotional liberation.

Emotional neglect as a child is a severe issue which can create painful emotional loneliness and also lead to long-term negative impacts on the person's choices regarding relationships and intimate partners and everything. In this book, you will learn a lot about toxic parenting and overcoming the results by establishing Boundaries, Reclaiming Your Emotional Autonomy, and Healing from Distant, Rejecting, Emotionally Immature Parents. This book is designed to help you understand the effects of toxic parenting and take essential steps to address the situation.

Toxic parenting can affect someone in different ways. Parents who are distant may have been physically present but emotionally unavailable, leaving children feeling isolated and ignored. Rejecting parents might have dismissed your feelings, criticized your achievements, or constantly compared you unfavorably to others. Self-involved parents, in contrast, were so caught up in their problems that they lacked the nurturing and direction you required.

This behavior pattern hurts the children's minds. It creates an environment where children start to believe that their needs and emotions are worthless and no one cares about them. The resulting emotional neglect can lead to profound and long-lasting effects. It can change your self-perspective and the interaction between you and others. With the impact of toxic parenting, you might often find yourself confused and seeking Validation from others, struggling with low self-esteem, or unable to trust your judgement.

The worst part of growing up in a toxic household is it does not end when you leave your childhood home. Because of the events you faced in your childhood, you might notice patterns that speak louder than words. For instance, you might be very much challenged to set personal boundaries, always put other people first, lack self-confidence and suffer from low self-esteem, among other things, which makes these toxic patterns act as barriers to establishing healthy relationships. Thus, the key message is to free yourself and the ones you care about from toxic parenting and start the healing process.

The most valuable actions to nurture oneself after toxic parenting are setting firm boundaries and regaining emotional independence. Maintaining healthy boundaries means protecting your emotional well-being and creating balanced relationships. Reclaiming your emotional autonomy means taking control of your feelings and reactions. These techniques will help you control your emotions while becoming an independent and healthy adult.

Overcoming the effects of toxic parenting is a process, a process that cannot be completed hastily but with time, effort, and understanding towards oneself. This is a roller coaster ride those entails accepting the fact that you've been hurt, comprehending how you've been mentally constituted by it, and then the process of rehabilitating and stepping forward. This book will guide you to a beautiful adult life full of confidence and no past trauma. You will understand how important self-care and self-compassion are and how to implement them. This task will involve identifying ways of dealing with negative feelings like anger and grief and positive thinking and attitudes about the self. Healing is also about accepting and being able to forgive – not precisely your parents, but yourself, for having thrived and enduring in that manner.

As you enter this healing process, knowing that you are not alone is helpful. Many people grew up with toxic parenting, and they face similar difficulties in adult life. Some of them are still suffering from the issue, some of them, like you, are trying to heal from the trauma, and some are already successful in healing themselves. This means that you are in a better position than those suffering. You are on the way to healing from the past trauma and successfully making your life, relationships, friendships and everything better. This book is written on my years of experience in helping people heal from their toxic parenting effects, and the strategies used in this book are tested and validated.

Along with the excellent part of healing from toxic parenting traumas, you also need to remember that this journey won't be easy. As past incidents already shape you, you must break and build a new, better and more successful version of yourself.

It's about time that you understand only you can liberate yourself from the shackles of toxic parenting and forge a positive, prosperous and joyful life. The boundaries, emotional independence, and self-healing should be worked through regarding personal and mutual relationships. This book is with you at every step of the journey, holding your hand, giving advice, cuddling, and kicking up the bum when needed! You are beginning the journey of healing and power for yourself. The time has come to stand up and take measures to achieve the life you want and deserve.

Chapter 1

Understanding Toxic Parenting

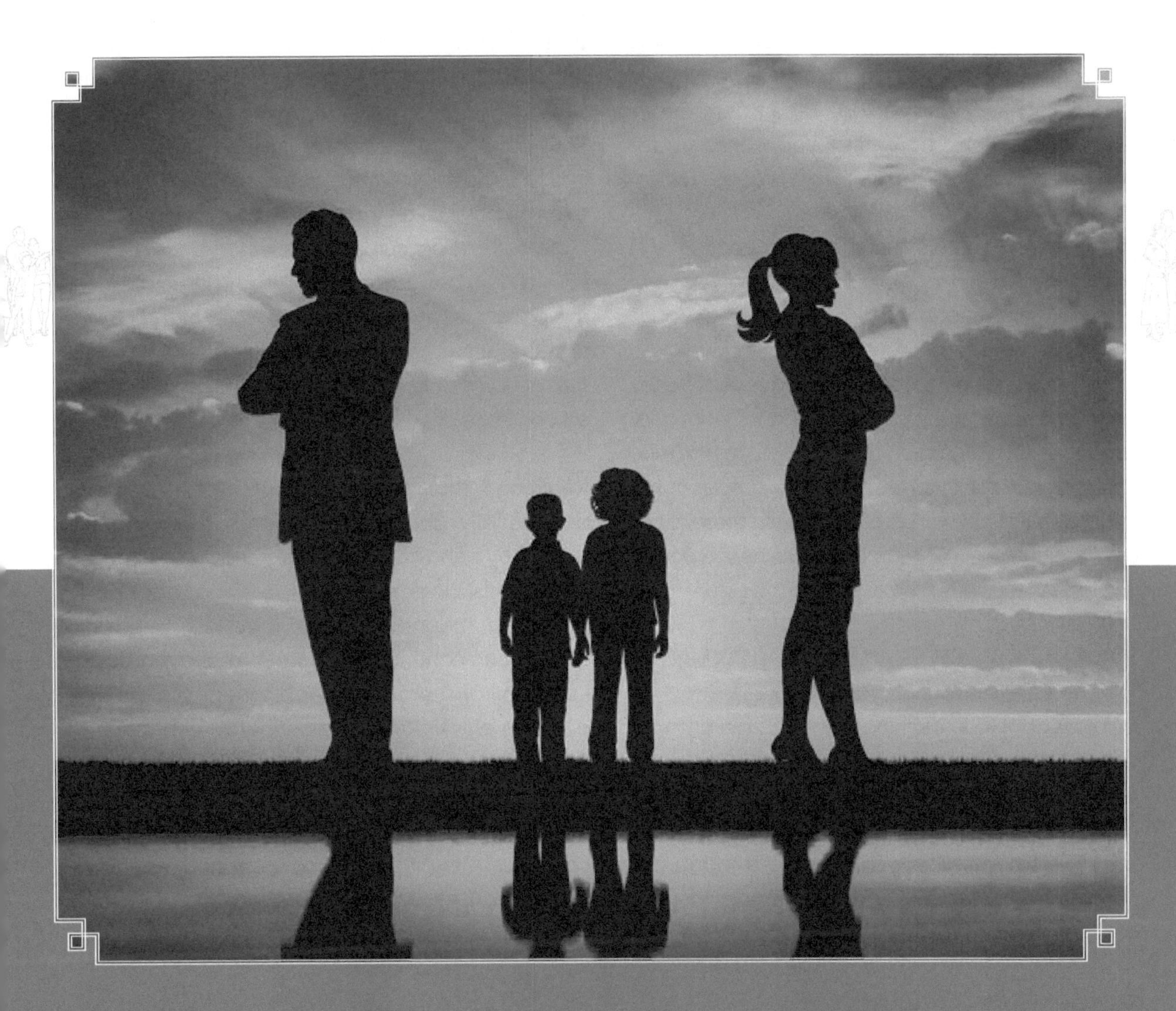

This is a very critical topic in the field of mental health, as it can affect someone for an extended period. Understanding toxic parenting is the very first step to healing from the wound you had as a child. It goes beyond mere recognition of harmful behaviors that can strongly affect someone's behaviors, mental health, and physical well-being. Understanding toxic parenting helps to break the cycle of abuse. It has been noticed that people who grew up with poisonous parents are at a high risk of running the same pattern in their relationships. By understanding toxic parenting, you can save your loved ones from the toxicity you went through. Everyone goes through different difficulties, but their solutions differ depending on the person. By understanding what kind of toxic parenting, you went through, you can choose the best healing process for you.

In this section, you will find different aspects of toxic parenting, and you will be enlightened on what toxic parenting entails and how to recognize poisonous parenting. This section consists of the knowledge on what a toxic parent is, typical tendencies of poisonous parents, effects of psychologically and emotionally toxic parents on grown-up children, realizing how much toxic parents affect you and real-life examples to help distinguish toxic behaviors of parents. All these factors are significant for your healing process, as you need to understand the cause before starting the cure.

What Makes a Parent Toxic?

It is essential to know what makes a parent toxic so that people can identify those who cause harm to their children. A toxic parent is one who negatively affects the psyche and sometimes the physical well-being of the child through their actions. These parents engage in behaviors that can be described as intrusive, oppressive, and toxic in terms of the impact they have on the child's self-esteem and psychological health.

When it comes to children, we are not only talking about their rights to have food, clothing, shelter, and protection from harm but also their rights to proper upbringing, care and support from their parents. In the absence of these basic needs and instead of their fulfilment, parents misuse substances and present their children with an environment in which an enriching life cannot be led. Such parenting styles lead to adverse psychological and emotional development, thus shaping a child's inability to form good relationships, lack of esteem, and low self-image.

Toxic parents infringe on this aspect of development in a way that makes children fear the world and puts them off balance on their own. Rather than being well protected and encouraged, children who toxic parents raise end up being worried, afraid and insecure about this position in society. Lack of security at home can adversely affect children's emotional and social growth, thus affecting different aspects such as performance in school and relationship issues.

Realizing that toxic parents do not just occasionally abuse their children or engage in unhealthy behaviors but consistently display these characteristics is critical to defining what toxic parenting means. Instead, they are behaviors that occur continually, characterize a particular individual or a group of people, negatively shape a child's emotions and psychology, contaminate that child's environment, and significantly hinder their recovery. The acknowledgement of toxic parents, or any abuse, sets the first stone in the process of mending a broken heart and healing for both the abused and the abusers.

People can deal with toxic products more suitably if they define the signs of toxic parenting. It enables them to go for counselling, group discussions, or any other assistance since it helps them start dealing with their feelings. It also allows them to know that false and abusive messages that were told to them as children stemmed from their parents' problems and not their worth or capability.

As a result, it is crucial to realize that toxic parenting is not simply several harmful actions but a particular pattern of interacting with children. Such behaviors may result from direct past experiences, trauma, mental illness, or other dysfunctional behavior models inherited by the parents. Also, through the realization of the root cause, people who suffer from toxic parenting can compassionately look at themselves as well as their parents and, most importantly, start the process of healing.

While evaluating what kind of parent is toxic, it is crucial to underline that recognizing these features does not mean a complete rejection of the parent as a person. Instead, it is the recognition of problematic behaviors and their effects. The separation of feelings toward parents, together with the necessity to change toxic behavior, can assist people with starting the process of wholeness and the actual transformation of their lives.

Finally, knowing what comprises a toxic parent is a significant milestone towards ending the abusive pattern and creating a healthy atmosphere for a person and generations to come. It includes not only awareness of toxic parent's hostile actions but also the attempts to actively change the situation and heal the one who went through it. In this way, people can regain their emotional independence, recover their self-esteem, and establish a base for better relations and a happier life.

Common Traits of Toxic Parents

It is essential to learn about the characteristics of toxic parents so it becomes easier to identify the experiences that may have shaped your life. These traits always result in emotional abuse, the destruction of one's self-esteem and the development of long-term relationship scars. Understanding these characteristics may help you begin to comprehend your experiences and work towards recovery.

MANIPULATION

Abuse can also take the form of toxicity, where parents engage in manipulation of their kids. This may range from guilt-tripping, emotional blackmail, and even the victim mentality. Possessive parents may, in one way or another, make their children feel they are the ones who influence or cause their parents joy or misfortune. This constant manipulation can damage the primary perception of the child, as well as cause significant instability in their psychological state, making them constantly feel guilty and inadequate as a child, as well as being solely responsible for their parent's feelings.

EMOTIONAL NEGLECT

In this case, the lack of proper response to the child's emotional needs by the parents is termed as emotional abuse. Of course, toxic parents may not be available orally, verbally, or emotionally as and when their child requires and deserves this from them. They can be inattentive to their children's feelings and needs, minimize or deny them, or sometimes cannot help soothe them. This is damaging because children grow up thinking they are unloved, unnoticed, and unheard, and this affects their entire personal development and self-esteem, as well as emotional stability in the future.

NARCISSISM

When parents are narcissistic, then they are self-absorbed individuals more concerned with their satisfaction, often to the detriment of their children. They may always require attention and praise, disregard other people's feelings and needs, and think they are superior to others. Narcissistic parents are often unkind, can pressure the child or children for the best performance and do not value or acknowledge children's accomplishments. This leads to an inferiority complex and the desperation for attention in their children.

CONTROL AND DOMINATION

Abusive parents are likely to be authoritatively controlling in the lives of their children; they decide things for them and prevent their children from being responsible for their actions. They could impose their beliefs and values to have their children think, feel, and behave in a specific manner with little chance to develop and make their own decisions. This may include behaviors as small as overseeing the other partner's tasks, setting particular expectations, or threats and punishments. Thus, they may experience poor problem-solving and low self-esteem in adulthood.

CRITICISM AND BLAME

Adverse treatment, especially scolding, is equivalent to toxicity in parenting. These parents commonly label their children by singling out their undesirable characteristics, failures and failures and disregarding the positives. They may turn around and accuse their children of being the cause of their miseries, or guilt and shame fill the atmosphere if their endeavors do not work out as intended. Such a barrage of criticism, as consistent and constant as it is, poses a risk to the child's self-esteem and even undermines their ability to have a cheerful disposition about them.

INCONSISTENT AND UNPREDICTABLE BEHAVIOR

Toxic parents may set limits or punish their children erratically, and this makes it unbearable for them to feel secure. They can flip from one polar behavior to another, and one can find them overbearing and affectionate at one time and either abusive or completely dismissive the next. Due to unpredictability, children may experience a lot of confusion and instability in their relationship with their parents, and their sole aim would be to shape themselves to fit their parent's unpredictable temperaments.

GASLIGHTING

The nature of gaslighting as a form of psychological abuse is that the toxic parent puts the child in doubt about their own experiences, memory, and even their mental stability. This can include negating events in front of the child when the child is observed to be telling a lie and turning facts around to make the youngster doubt what is real. Considering the above effects, it can be ascertained that gaslighting hinders the development of a child's confidence, creates confusion in their ability to understand and interpret reality, and poses a significant danger to their perceiving sense of self and self-identity.

Identifying these general characteristics of toxic parents is the way to begin the process of experiencing the effects that have been created. It helps to open one's eyes to forms of abuse that might have become naturalized in one's family of origin and to start the process of recovery of one's emotional agency. With this in mind, you can create new boundaries with others, practice more self-compassion, and strive for better relationships.

The Psychological and Emotional Impact on Adult Children

The various effects of toxic parents on the psychological and emotional well-being of their children are apparent if they were indulged as they were growing up. These are important because they can affect the clients' perception of themselves, their interpersonal relationships, and their overall health conditions. It is essential to acknowledge and learn about these effects to identify and overcome obstacles that such experiences create for one to begin the process of recovery and improvement.

1. LOW SELF-ESTEEM

The first psychological impact of growing up with toxic parents is that one may suffer from reduced self-worth. Verbal abuse, insults, and emotional abuse of any sort make the adult offspring feel unlovable and incompetent. This means they may learn negative parental messages and constantly believe they are inadequate. This poor self-image will extend into all facets of the person's life, including career choice, relationships with others, and effective pursuit of desirable roles and objectives.

2. ANXIETY AND DEPRESSION

These toxic behaviors make the environment unpredictable, and this aspect alone leads to anxiety and depression. Some of the general fear states that adult children may go through include protracted worry, fear of failure, and symptoms of sadness or hopelessness. The arduous emotional labor of meeting the expectations and regulating the parent's mood informs persistent anxiety, whereas the lack of recognition and comforting signals fosters hopelessness.

3. DIFFICULTY SETTING BOUNDARIES

Another exciting aspect mentioned is that many adult children were raised in families where boundaries were not an option and thus struggled to establish proper boundaries in adulthood. They may need help to refuse a request or to express and demand their rights to 'own space,' for instance. This results in them being exploitable, overwhelmed, and lacking self-determination in their relationships and careers.

4. TRUST ISSUES

Toxic parents engage in the process of misleading and confusing a child in areas such as trust, and this is because toxic parents are hypocrites. This is why adult children may struggle to trust others; they always feel like they will be betrayed or rejected. One might refrain from starting new relationships, consistently doubt others' intentions, or have problems with closeness. Such suspicion can help them develop effective social relations but may force them to remain isolated and lonely as they cannot establish close relationships.

5. PERFECTIONISM AND FEAR OF FAILURE

A common coping strategy that arises from growing up with toxic parents is perfectionism, given the effort to please the parents in a bid to avoid ridicule. They may also have high self-expectations; they may become very hard critics when they cannot meet them. This perfectionism can be crippling and results in a non-imposter refusing to take on a project that might be challenging in the fear that they might fail. That constant pressure to perform can also lead the employee to burnout or the feeling that they can never do enough.

6. CODEPENDENCY

This is something that takes place in many adult

children as they were raised under toxic parents. They may have learnt to make others happy at the expense of their happiness, always looking for value in caretaker and people-pleasing roles. This can lead to the creation of skewed and problematic roles in interpersonal relationships wherein they are automatically seen as the ones who must also care for people's moods. Codependency results in hostility, the feeling of being drained, and a failure to manage an individual's own needs and self-development.

7. EMOTIONAL DYSREGULATION

Another unbeneficial behavior of such parents is that they do not teach their children how to manage their emotions appropriately, and growing up with such parents makes it hard for adult children to regulate their emotions. They might display obsessions with rage, mood swings, frustration issues, or be unable to manage or adequately express emotions. These changes affect their relationships, work, and daily living capacity, making it hard to manage stress and conflicts.

8. RELATIONSHIP CHALLENGES

The relational patterns established with toxic parents often carry over into adult relationships. Adult children may have difficulty in forming intimate relationships, have fears of abandonment, or may choose a partner who behaves in the same way as their parents did. They might end up choosing partners that are either abusive or, in some other way, unhealthy, thus reproducing the hostile environment of their childhoods. They could also completely shut down any form of relationship for fear of having the raw wounds of a previous relationship re-opened.

Understanding the Impact of Toxic Parenting

Toxic parenting can influence an individual's life in the worst way; their personalities are defiled, and what they experience impacts their mental health, emotions, and social life. The effects of such parenting styles tend to be lifelong; they shape the developing child's perception of self and the world. Identifying and analyzing such effects is essential to severing toxic ties and working to become healthier individuals.

SELF-IDENTITY AND SELF-WORTH

Generally, toxic parenting affects perception and how one sees oneself. Verbal abuse, anger, and lack of trust affect a person and make them feel inadequate and unworthy. The children who grow up in such homes may buy into hopeless attitudes about themselves and thus feel incompetent and undeserving. Therefore, they may face significant issues, such as low self-esteem, lack of confidence, and a shattered sense of self-identification as they grow up. Regaining one's confidence requires overcoming these cognitions and replacing them with realistic, benevolent perceptions of the self.

EMOTIONAL AND PSYCHOLOGICAL HEALTH

The effects of toxic parents on the child's emotional and psychological well-being can be experienced in several forms. Numerous adult children have been described as suffering from anxiety, depression and other related conditions that are chronic. These chronic stressors arising from adverse interactions with a toxic parent may raise the level of threat perception and general anxiety disorders. Further on, there is an absence of affection and approval. Consequently, the individual can experience a void and isolation and even see signs of depression in front of him. Solving these challenges implies professional therapy to deal with and recover from various traumas experienced.

ATTACHMENT AND RELATIONSHIP PATTERNS

A person has various attachment styles that are shaped during childhood and define further behavioral patterns regarding relationships. By toxic parenting, children develop insecure styles of attachment, including anxious, avoidant, or disorganized attachment. Adults with such attachment styles may encounter problems in trusting, intimacy and identifying the appropriate boundary line in any relationship. They might find themselves repeating toxic patterns with partners, friends, or even their children. Developing secure attachment involves learning to trust, communicate effectively, and establish healthy boundaries.

COPING MECHANISMS AND DEFENSE STRATEGIES

These children have most certainly learned ways of dealing with toxic parents, as well as strategies to protect themselves from their hostile home environments. Some of these could be repression, approval-seeking, obsession for order and cleanliness, or even repression. Although these behaviors may be functional in childhood, they are often considered dysfunctional in adulthood and impede the healthy development of one's emotions and self-sufficiency skills. This means that to overcome these unhelpful ways of behaving, one has to learn healthier ways of dealing with stress and managing one's emotions.

FEAR OF CONFLICT AND AVOIDANCE BEHAVIORS

Adult children of toxic parents suffer from an increased level of anxiety, and especially, they avoid conflict. They might avoid confrontation to the end as they fear the reaction that always followed quarrels in their childhood. This may lead to passive aggression, unspoken anger or inability to speak up for oneself and or express one's needs. It is a healthy skill to learn how to deal with conflict in a way that helps a person and their relationship to grow.

Real-life Stories: Recognizing Toxic Behavior in Parents

The following is a collection of stories from people who have been exposed to toxic parents, showing how to spot and comprehend these behaviors. These scenarios expose a reminder of the ordeals faced by adult kids from toxic parents and, by extension, the need to validate such concerns to foster healthy well-being.

SARAH'S STORY: THE PERILS OF PERFECTIONISM

Sarah has lived in a home where nothing she did was appropriate or to the standard expected of her. For example, her mother is a perfectionist who used to scold her for her work, state her mistakes and demand more. 'Even when I scored 95% on a test, my mother was bound to ask why I did not score 100%,' says Sarah. This made it relentless and, in due course, put a lot of pressure on Sarah to the extent that she got severe anxiety and an obsession with perfection. It was only as a grown woman that she suffered from constant stress and exhaustion due to the pressure that she was putting on herself to meet unreasonably high expectations. Sarah could work out that she is not perfect and develop an ability to accept everything about her during therapy. In this series, she has learnt to accept success as usual without that circle's constant search for approval.

TOM'S STORY: EMOTIONAL NEGLECT AND ITS LINGERING EFFECTS

Tom's father did not care for or express affection towards him and was disinterested in the events of his life. Tom speaks about when he has never heard his father tell him he loved or was proud of him. Such psychiatric abuse made Tom feel that he was not worthy of being seen and treated as a worthy human being. He struggled to build good relationships and intimacy, especially in adulthood, just in case he was rejected, like how he felt during childhood. Tom was a patient who suffered from depression and loneliness for many years, and he finally came to therapy. He was able to accept one's feelings in the relationship and look for loving relationships where he would be welcomed. Tom's journey towards healing involved building a supportive network of friends who provided the emotional connection he had longed for.

LINDA'S STORY: THE MANIPULATIVE PARENT

One of the main issues in the story is the bad behavior of Linda's mother, who was an abusive woman who manipulated her children. Linda says: 'She would force us to perform specific tasks for her in an almost manipulative way, making us feel as if we are to blame for her discomfort. This manipulation made Linda feel always that she was not adequate and brought anxiety into her life. In her adult life, she would have codependency issues where she would always place the needs of others before her own. Although Linda learned manipulative patterns from her mother, by the time she realized the problem, she sought the help of a therapist to set some boundaries. She also managed to understand her own needs and how to deal with pathological ones in other people. Linda now looks for healthy self-care and only includes individuals who accept her freedom.

EMILY'S STORY: OVERCOMING GASLIGHTING

Emily's father, like many abusers, was a master of gaslighting: he would twist the facts to make Emily doubt her perception or her memory of an event." He would deny things that happened, making me feel like I was going crazy," Emily shows. This manipulation led to the grounding, conflict in one's head and full-blown Modern Day Self Doubt. It can be concluded that throughout the latter part of her life, Emily was characterized by indecision and a lack of trust in her judgment. With the assistance of a knowledgeable therapist, she started to understand the nature of the abusive behavior of her father, including gaslighting. Emily's problems in this story show that one needs to learn to trust their intuition and acknowledge what is happening to them. She now feels surer about her decisions and better understands what is real.

The following real-life stories present the multiple and severe consequences of a toxic upbringing. They also state that it is crucial to identify such behaviors and visit a specialist to prevent their impacts from continuing. Recovery entails focusing on the abuse and its effects on the heart and mind, as well as gaining knowledge regarding better ways of relating and creating healthier boundaries. Hence, therapy, reflection and overall support from society and other recovery fellowship organizations are helpful platforms that can assist a person to extricate themself from the poisonous cycle and bring a positive change into their life.

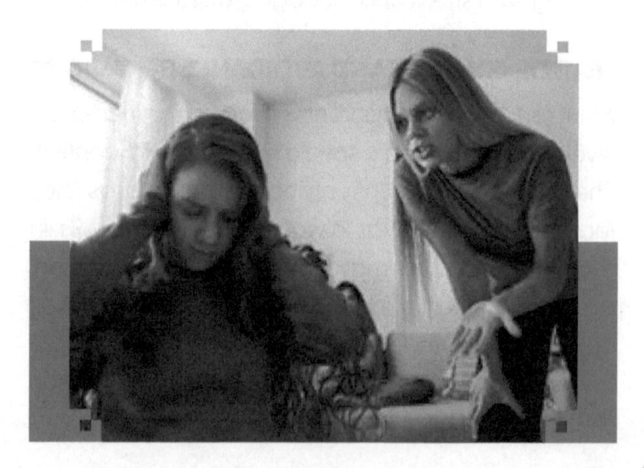

Chapter 2

Types of Toxic Parents

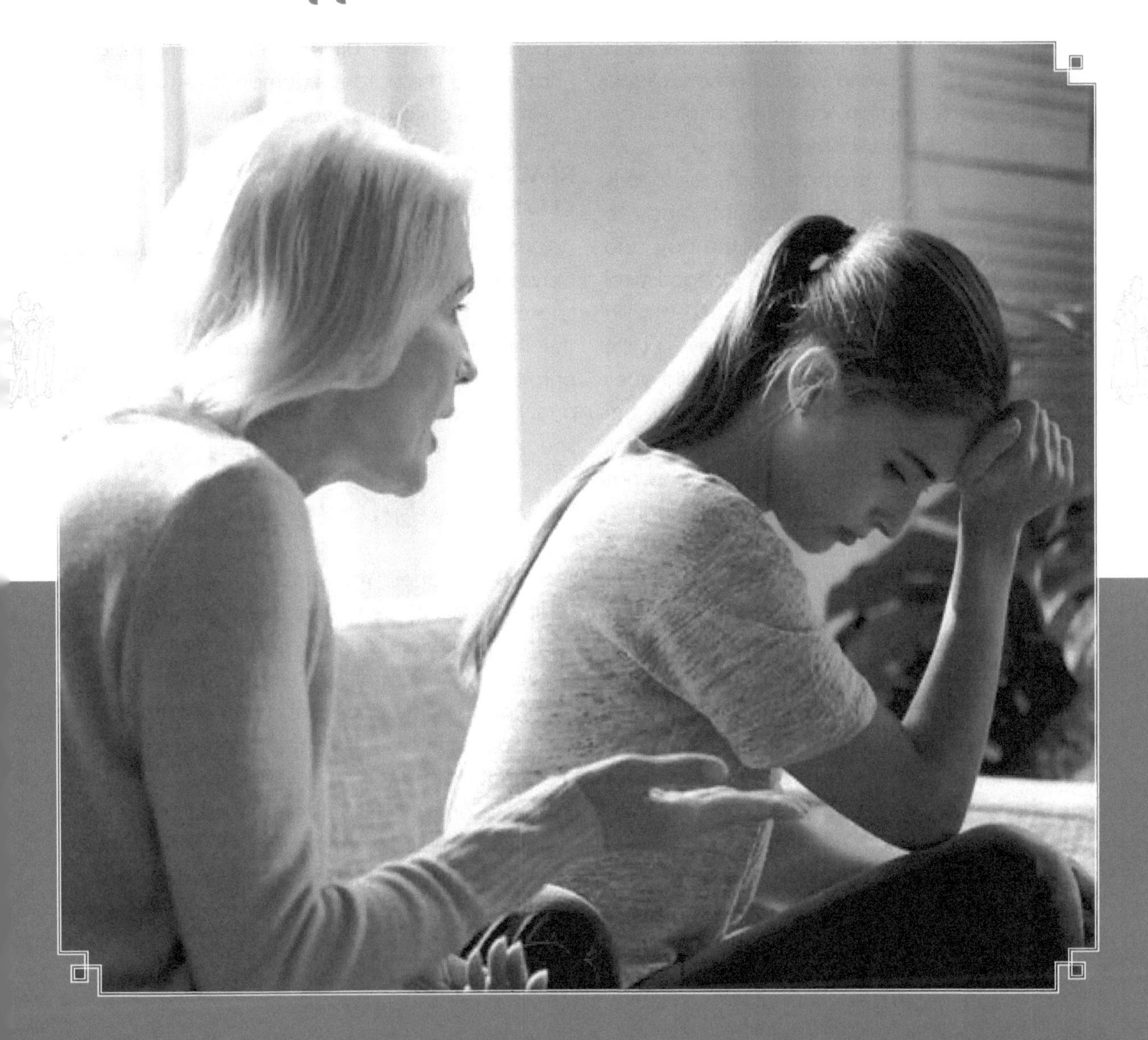

Toxic parenting manifests in various ways, each with distinct methods that shape the type of poisonous parent. Understanding these types can illuminate the toxic mechanisms and provide insights into overcoming these traumas. Here, we explore different types of toxic parents, their behaviors, coping mechanisms, and examples to illustrate these concepts with emotional depth

The Narcissistic Parent

- Characteristics and Behaviors: Narcissistic parents are always in their world with an uncontrollable urge to get admiration, and they neglect the emotions of their children. They might:
- Demand Constant Attention and Praise: It is like the child going home all bright, ready to enumerate their achievements of the day, and the parent drowns the child with their egotistical accomplishments. Everything the child accomplishes is downplayed, and they feel like they do not matter. For instance, if a child goes to school and comes back with an award, the parent will, instead of appreciating the child, tell them, 'When I was your age, I got double what you have got, and you have not tried enough'.
- Use Manipulation to Maintain Control: A narcissistic parent will say to the child, 'If you loved me, you would do this for me,' thereby putting the child in a self-ensnaring bind because they cannot break away without feeling guilty. This might include the parent making the child feel they are a terrible child simply because they do not obey the parent's decision, which could be to stay home when the child wants to go out.
- Dismiss or Invalidate Their Child's Feelings and Needs: This is because a narcissistic parent negates the child's feelings when they utter feelings such as, "You have no right to feel like that." For instance, if a child is bullied at school and comes home feeling sad, instead of comforting the child, the parent may tell them, "You're only doing this for attention."
- Display Grandiosity and a Sense of Entitlement: They want to be pampered and focus only on their side of the story. This shapes the child's development by receiving the idea of being existent merely to provide for the parent or have the parent provide for them. Such an example could be a parent predicting that the child must leave all their engagements and attend to the parent's demands regardless of what the child was overseeing.

REACT POORLY TO CRITICISM OR PERCEIVED SLIGHTS:

An unfavorable comment or feeling of rejection may lead to anger, and the child learns that speaking the truth is wrong. For example, while the child articulates a complex scenario that portrays the parent as unfair, the parent could get angry and respond with words like, "How dare you speak to me like that, you ungrateful kid."

Coping Strategies

- Set Boundaries: You should know for yourself what kinds of behaviors are acceptable and what behaviors are unaccepted. For instance, if your parents call you and immediately yell at you to come and attend to them, tell them, "I require my space at the moment, and thus cannot attend to you.
- Limit Contact: Minimize contacts to guard against stress for employees. This may entail reducing the frequency of calls or shortening visits and other interactions conducted with healthy-sounding volunteers. For instance, if a visit takes a digressing toll on the person's

emotional intelligence, it is advisable to end the visit by saying, "I have to go now, but we could continue this conversation later.

- Seek Validation Elsewhere: The best thing is that they establish close friends and mentors who can provide genuine appreciation and encouragement. This may be as basic as dialing a friend's number after an episode with your parents to speak on your grievances.
- Therapy: Consult with a counsellor to deal with self-esteem problems and acquire skills in dealing with its implications, understanding the importance of acknowledging one's feelings. It is revealed that therapy can serve as the place to decipher your emotions and the ways to construct more beneficial and adequate patterns of conduct.

The Controlling Parent

- Understanding Control Mechanisms: The parents chloroform their children and make them allow the parents to make all the decisions on the children's behalf. They might:
- Micromanage Daily Activities and Decisions: Consider a mother or a father deciding what his or her child will wear, play with, or with whom to make friends, or even what activities the child may engage in during his or her free time; all these leave the child with no say. For instance, one can force the choice of an outfit for the next day; thus, the child has no say in it.
- Use Guilt and Fear to Influence Behavior: Statements such as "If you don't do as I say, you'll regret it" instill fear and subordination in individuals. For example, a parent can tell a child, "If you do not study this subject, you will be jobless in future, and you will be a letdown to me.
- Undermine Self-Confidence by Questioning Abilities: It reduces the child's self-esteem to the extent that they start doubting their capacity to make any decision. An example is a parent who, each time the child errs, will say, "You are such a mess; you cannot do anything right."

Actions to Take to Get One's Freedom Back

- Assert Independence: Learn to make choices and stick with them no matter what, even if you are mocked for them. For example, deciding to follow one's passion rather than what their parents have set for them, such as choosing art over law.
- Establish Boundaries: The time and effort one is willing to give must be stated and enforced. For instance, "Thank you for your concern, though I must do this alone."
- Seek Support: Get to know other mothers going through the same experience, seek advice, and get motivated by them. For example, going for a session of an association of CoDA – controlling parents – adult children association.

The Emotionally Immature Parent

Identifying Emotional Immaturity

Emotionally immature parents struggle with managing their own emotions and often react childishly. They might:

- Overreacting to Minor Issues: A child could easily get frightened by an ow coming down while drinking some fluid and make an exaggerated response such as flailing the arms; the child could easily spill the liquid, thereby increasing the chances of signaling to the ow that something is wrong. For instance, a parent may shout at a child when they make a small mess on the table, which makes the child so afraid of compounding the mistake made by making even a bigger one.

- Avoid Responsibility and Blame Others: If the child is presented with issues, they will blame others and thus learn that responsibility should not be addressed. For instance, a parent may find fault in his or her child and tell him or her, "You are the one who made me a sad mother/father."
- Struggle with Empathy and Emotional Support: They cannot deal with physical affection, which their child requires, let alone psychological support, which the child receives in the form of invalidation or complete disregard. For instance, if a child loses a best friend through a fight, the parent uses phrases such as "You will get over it; it is not that serious."
- Exhibit Unpredictable Moods and Behavior: The child is left very insecure, always having to tread very carefully for fear of what the parent might do next; this makes the child very insecure. For instance, a parent will be soft-spoken at one point and then become enraged at the next without apparent cause.

BUILDING EMOTIONAL RESILIENCE

- Self-Education: Education concerning the nature of healthy emotions and managing anger. Remember that your parent's reaction must be expected as it is generated from their problems, not your worth. It is helpful to read books related to EI and personal maturity.
- Develop Emotional Awareness: a. Acknowledge and affirm your emotions, saying they are acceptable to feel this way. This could be writing down the feelings one experiences daily to accept those feelings.
- Self-Care: Do things that make your heart happy- write down your thoughts, exercise, contemplate or do any other activity you like. For example, spend some time daily engaging in an activity that sustains you.
- Therapeutic Support: Fill therapy sessions to learn how to counter/manage emotional problems and improve an emotional life. Counselling for anxiety can assist a person in regaining healthy ways of thinking and coping with stress.

The Abusive Parent

Forms of Abuse: Physical, Emotional, Verbal

Abusive parents inflict harm through various forms, each leaving deep scars:

- Physical Abuse: Physical violence, such as hitting or slapping, only increases fear and physical pain in an ecosystem. For instance, a parent corrects a child physically, thus creating fear and trauma in them.
- Emotional Abuse: Looking at the nature of ill-treatment, it can be noted that they all work to unrecognize the child and cause severe emotional harm. The emotionally abusive parent may continuously humiliate the child by using words such as 'You are useless' 'and You always get it wrong'.
- Verbal Abuse: Verbal abuse includes insults, actual and implied threats, and biting criticism, which are not only psychologically abusive but also inflict a detailed and calculated assault on a child's self-image and sense of security. For instance, a parent who frequently yells and makes statements that other people of the child's gender are better than the child or deserve better than the child will make the child feel scared and worthless.

HEALING FROM ABUSE

- Acknowledge the Abuse: Acknowledge and agree to the fact that the abuse happened, but it was not you're doing. This might involve telling yourself, "What was done to me was wrong, and I did not have a hand in it."

- Safety First: Make sure you are physically located out of harm's way from the person abusing you. This might mean escaping to another room or standing across from your partner. For example, fleeing from an abusive partner or severing ties with the abusive partner. Friends and family.
- Therapy: Undergo counselling with a professional that focuses on trauma to work through the effect of the abuse in regaining any damaged self-esteem and safety. Counseling can enable an individual to come to terms with their emotions, thus attaining better ways of positive thinking and behaving.
- Build a Support Network: So, there should be people around who would love for you and support you all the time. This could mean it will be in a support group for abused women or relying on close friends or family.

The Distant or Rejecting Parent

Effects of Emotional Neglect

Distant or rejecting parents fail to provide the emotional support and connection children need, leading to:

- Feelings of Unworthiness and Rejection: Children grow up thinking they are unimportant and unwanted, automatically making them doubt their existence. For instance, a child may develop an idea that they are not worthy of the parent's time or attention, resulting in low self-esteem.
- Difficulty Forming Secure Attachments: Without a model for healthy attachment, the child struggles to form secure relationships. This might manifest in adult relationships where the person has trouble trusting others or fears intimacy.
- Chronic Loneliness and Emotional Voids: The lack of emotional connection leaves a deep void, fostering loneliness and isolation. For instance, they may feel a persistent emptiness and long for meaningful connections.

STRATEGIES FOR SELF-COMPASSION AND HEALING

- Practice Self-Compassion: Do not judge or scold yourself for how you feel because these are genuine emotions. Such as: 'I will comfort myself with positive statements such as 'I deserve love and care.'
- Build Healthy Relationships: Look for and cultivate a nurturing and understanding person to get the lacking affection. This could include coming out to make friends that accept one or joining groups of people with similar interests as that of the individual.
- Therapy: Enter counselling to talk about the feelings of being undeserving and begin the process of learning self-nurturing the same way you were starved of love. At therapeutic levels, you will be able to understand and recover from the effects of emotional abandonment, thus developing a healthy self-perception.
- Mindfulness and Self-Care: Participate in practices that build up even, gain and knowledge about yourself. For instance, mindfulness meditation can be used to be aware and stay engaged with one's feelings.
- Awareness of these toxic parents and their characteristic behaviors is the first step to coming to terms with their role in one's life. When using such coping mechanisms and attempting to get help, one has the chance to start overcoming past violations and have a better life. I want you to know that healing is long and gradual, and every path you take is essential.

Chapter 3

Recognizing the Effects on Your Life

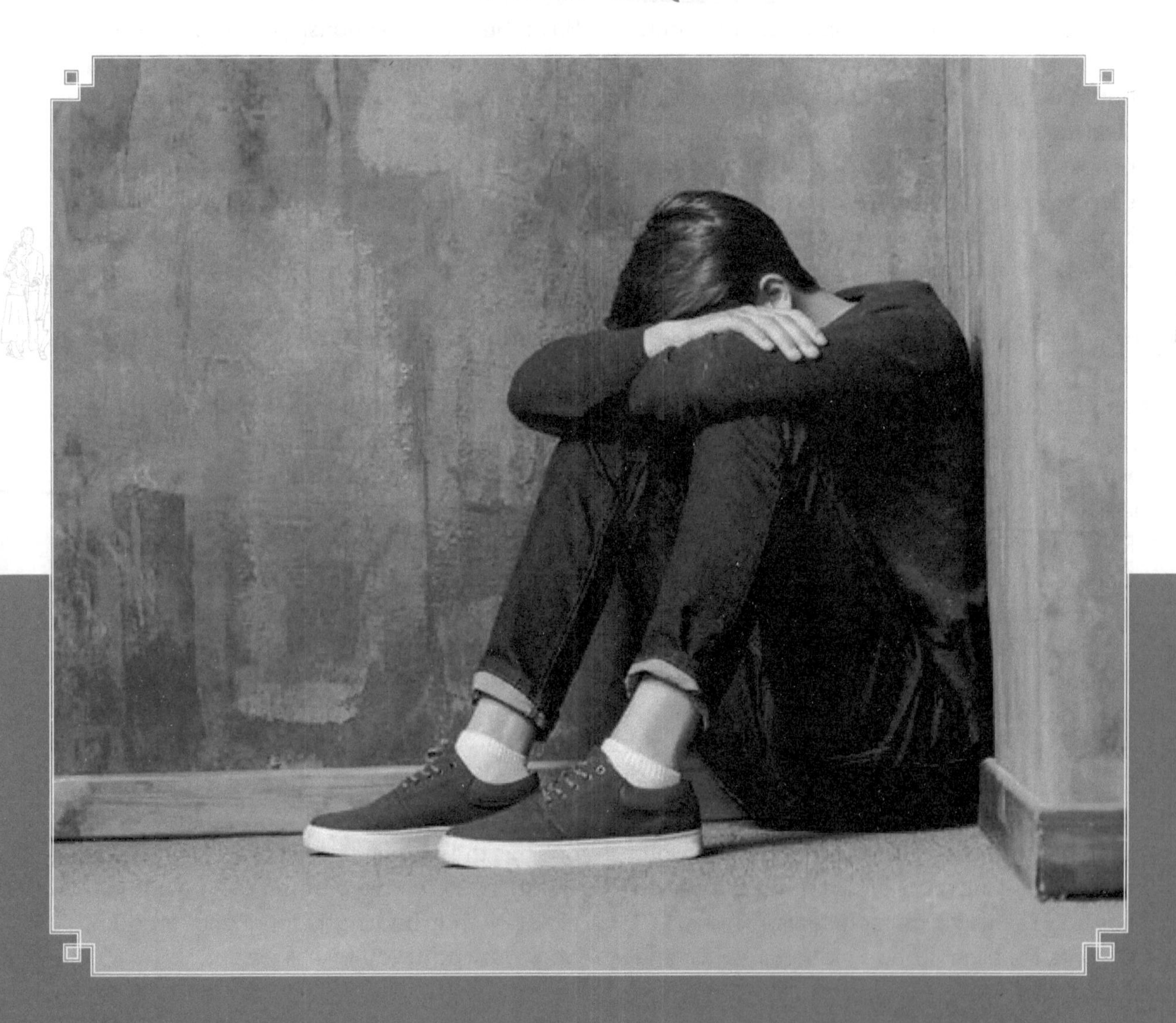

Toxic parenting does not simply affect one's childhood; it deeply imprints on one's psyche and influences how one forms self-identity and interactions with others and the environment. It is critical to comprehend and acknowledge these effects and pressures; this knowledge will allow you to work through the problems that impede your recovery. This way, you can take control of the toxic environment, receiving the necessary information to escape it and establish a healthier life.

It is vital to know how toxic parents affect your life to regain your emotional health and take control of your life. Maltreatment in childhood has a very long-lasting effect on the psychological well-being of the person long after childhood has been left far behind. These effects can, in turn, be presented in forms such as body image disturbances and troubled interpersonal and identity issues.

Realizing these effects is the starting point for addressing the issue. By recognizing these patterns of toxic parenting, one can change the poisonous patterns deliberately. This aspect assists in explaining why one may experience problems like low self-esteem, perfectionism, or relationship problems.

It provides clarity and validation for your experiences, allowing you to separate your self-worth from the negative influences of your past.

This recognition is crucial for breaking negative cycles. Toxic parenting shapes toxic patterns of cognition and behavior that can be passed from one generation to another if they are not treated. Understanding these patterns and appreciating the chances, you help them change for the company's benefit. This may consist of questioning one's mental patterns, changing coping strategies that are dysphoric, and learning new patterns of communicating with people.

Once you know the impacts, social validation also enables you to seek the best help and treatment. The 'therapeutic infrastructure', whether from trained professionals – therapists and support groups – or self-helpers, allows one to use appropriate instruments if/when the source of pain is discerned. It also suggests that there can be more significant results to the attempts at healing emotional pain and developing coping mechanisms when a focus is placed on certain types of patients.

It is relevant to recognize how toxic parents affected one's life to have realistic expectations as to personal healing. One should incredibly stress that healing from such profound dysfunctions is lengthy. Knowing your experiences makes you sober and patient with your journey.

This awareness helps enhance relations with other people. The effects highlighted here are self, difference, and relationship. This means that if the reader understands how toxic parenting functions within their interactions, they can start changing the scripts of relationships. It assists in clearly defining what is expected in a relationship and avoiding unhealthy relationships with toxic people.

In summary, awareness of the consequences of toxic parents helps create a framework for restoring emotional state and personality. It provides you with the understanding to deal with past traumas, question negative thinking patterns, and develop new patterns of interaction with yourself and others. All of this makes self-awakening and understanding of one's situation crucial in escaping toxic patterns laid by parents and transitioning into a healthier life.

Identifying Toxic Patterns in Your Behavior

Realising unhealthy behavior and changing the dynamics of toxic patterns are two ways by which emotional sovereignty can be achieved. As such, it can be difficult but, at the same time, rewarding for adult children of toxic parents to identify these patterns in themselves. This is a process where one must be aware and considerate of oneself, look at certain feelings, attitudes, and behaviors and trace their origins. In this section, it is necessary to describe toxic patterns that might appear and present approaches to their recognition and regulation.

1. SELF-SABOTAGE

That is why self-sabotage is one of the common patterns stemming from beliefs formed during childhood. Suppose you catch yourself sabotaging your success in relationships, job, and personal development. In that case, you might subconsciously say to yourself that you do not deserve success and happiness. For example, postposing activities, continuous wavering or setting very high goals that one cannot achieve are self-sabotaging behaviors.

To address self-sabotage:
Examine Triggers: Find out the triggers of self-destructive behaviors. Is there another time in weekly or daily cycles that appears to be the stimulus for these patterns?

Challenge Negative Beliefs: Consider where these beliefs come from and what they are based on, then question them. These beliefs should not be our beliefs about ourselves.

Set Realistic Goals: Set realistic targets and work towards them while making little party wins because the mindset loves to sabotage.

2. PEOPLE-PLEASING

Blameful behavior may manifest itself in people-pleasing since this behavior is caused by a need for recognition and fear of rejection, which can be rooted in toxic communication between parents. If you always put the needs and wants of others before yours, or if you find yourself agreeing to do things you do not like because you do not want to let others down, then you are probably a people-pleaser.

To address people-pleasing:
Assert Your Needs: Practice assertiveness by clearly communicating your needs and boundaries. Start with small steps to build confidence.

Self-Reflection: Reflect on why you need to please others and its impact on your well-being. Is this behavior rooted in fear of rejection or a need for validation?

Seek Balance: Strive to balance accommodating others and caring for yourself. It's essential to recognize that your needs are valid and deserve attention.

3. OVER-APOLOGIZING

There is always a time when one has to apologize, but if one is continuously tendering an apology, then this shows that they are always overly guilty, even when there is no need for it. If you catch yourself apologizing often, and not only when it is necessary or it is appropriate to do so – this can indicate that you are a chronic apologist, i.e., you are used to taking on much more blame than deserved based on the misunderstanding of responsibility for others' reactions.

To address over-apologizing:
Assess the Situation: Thus, one should first assess the degree to which an apology is appropriate before using this interpersonal communication strategy. Are you genuinely guilty of an offence, or are you just sorry for the heck of it?

Practice Self-Compassion: Pronounce forgiveness as it is okay to make human mistakes and may not necessarily need an apology.

Set boundaries: Accept your rights within certain relationships and situations, as every person has them. This is how effective assertiveness is and how different it is from aggression. Realize that being an assertive person and defending yourself does not make you a wicked person.

4. AVOIDANCE OF CONFLICT

Non-assertiveness is one of the defence mechanisms that may be formed in response to an emotional condition in childhood that can be characterized as being without order or containing many conflicts. If you find yourself avoiding conflict or situations requiring you to stand up for yourself, you may be a conflict-avoidant person.

To address conflict avoidance:
Identify Fear: Explore the underlying fears associated with conflict. Are you afraid of criticism, rejection, or escalation of disputes?

Build Communication Skills: Ensure appropriate ways and means of communication to solve interpersonal conflicts to develop the best solution. Be conscious of how you regularly communicate your thoughts and feelings with others.

Face Conflicts Gradually: To overcome this problem, one should begin with comparatively easy conflicts so that, succeeding at them, they will gain confidence and gradually work their way up to more complicated conflicts.

5. OVERDEPENDENCE ON OTHERS FOR VALIDATION

Suppose one continually looks to others for reinforcement to feel good about oneself. In that case, there might not be any healthy self-esteem that has developed in adulthood due to toxic rearing. This overdependence can sometimes give the person unstable self-esteem, and they cannot make independent decisions independently.

To address overdependence on others for validation:
Develop Self-Awareness: Self-reflecting means knowing your value and worth regardless of what others may say about you.

Build Self-Esteem: Promote behaviors and actions that foster self-esteem and promote worth in children and young people. When achieving individual targets, set personal goals and also rejoice over the achievements made.

Cultivate Internal Validation: There is validation by acknowledging and supporting internal approval by affirming one's success and ability. Practice self-acceptance and self-compassion.

Changing destructive behaviors and personal habits is not easy; it takes time and effort, and every individual must be willing to improve. Therefore, an awareness of these patterns and taking active measures to change or overcome them is not only the process of 'banishing the demons of the past and healing the self' but is creating a path to a better life. It is now essential to know that change is not a one-day process; therefore, it's good to encourage yourself and be patient with yourself.

The Impact on Self-Esteem and Self-Worth

Toxic parenting can rank itself as one of the most influential factors in a person's life. These toxic behaviors that these parents exhibit affect their self-esteem and self-worth, thus experiencing hardship in their adulthood. Here are a few long-term Hopelessness, low Self-Esteem and Self-Worth due to toxic parenting.

RELATIONSHIP DIFFICULTIES

People who become toxic parents develop relationship issues, especially as adults. They need help to build proper relationships. They may need help concerning trust in relationships, independence, and assertiveness. This can easily lead to more unhealthy relationships and, therefore, more feelings of unworthiness. The constant fear of rejection and the entrenched notion of undeserving love and respect make working on and maintaining relationships difficult. Subsequently, such people might end up with other individuals and stay in relationships which are as toxic as those they experienced in their childhood.

PROFESSIONAL CHALLENGES

Low self-esteem significantly affects career choices and professional growth. People who had toxic parents as children may lack confidence in their abilities, so why venture? They may feel that they need more success. This kind of self-doubt can lead to the symptoms of underachievement or the tendency to take the absolute worst of what one deserves; this is because the individual can avoid situations that they believe they deserve. After all, their potential can be questioned. This becomes especially apparent when such women suffer from the fear of failure as well as low self-esteem as they retreat from self-advocacy, promotions, or career-switching. They pointed out how this professional stagnation affects their economic status and solidifies the negative perceptions that individuals with such characteristics have about themselves.

MENTAL HEALTH ISSUES

Thus, the actualization of low self-esteem and self-worth is associated with mental health issues, including depression, anxiety, and stress. A person finds solutions for the negative beliefs that get internalized from childhood, which is why they continue experiencing emotional and psychological problems. The patient can feel hopeless and helpless and think that life is not worth living. It is for these reasons that these mental health challenges can become severe, reducing the quality of life and limiting the patient's functionality in day-to-day activities. Psychological exertion may also cause bodily health issues in conjunction with other psychological pressures adversely affecting their health.

SELF-SABOTAGE

People with low self-esteem are likely to think and act negatively, such as bringing the task to the last moment, avoiding it entirely or using substances. These behaviors can cause the clients to fail and thus strengthen negative notions about themselves. While they continue to procrastinate and avoid tasks, it simply means they are afraid of being unable to do something right and end up with lost opportunities and dreams. As for one of the patterns of self-destruction, substance abuse can take its place as well; although it can be an attempt to escape one's suffering, it does not work and only digs a deeper hole. Self-destructiveness seriously interferes with individual and career development and maintains a negative perspective on the probability of achievement or their capacity to be happy.

SOCIAL WITHDRAWAL

Poor self-esteem also leads to withdrawal and rejection from community life. Some adults may withdraw from society because they fear what people say about them or may not want to mingle with people for several reasons, thus leading to the isolation of the patients. This tends to make the patients feel lonely and can worsen their condition, causing incredibly depressed and anxious patients. It isolates people from others and does not allow them to do things that will assist in building up one's character and developing self-confidence to enable them to come out of the cage.

DIFFICULTY ACCEPTING COMPLIMENTS

People with low self-esteem have difficulty receiving compliments or positive remarks as they nearly reject them. They can easily underestimate themselves or give little credit to their accomplishments, arguing that it was easy or that they were lucky. This capacity to fail in internalizing positive messages custodies their negative self-esteem and does not percolate them to construct a healthy self-regard. This also affects their interaction with others, and they may be rude or indifferent when receiving compliments.

CHRONIC GUILT AND SHAME

There is also the tension of Guilt and shame experienced by adults who have low self-esteem. Therapists reckoned that the patients of such parents could experience a continual sense of Guilt due to their inability to make their parents proud or fulfil the perceived inadequacies of their lives. A lasting feeling of Guilt emerges that results in self-punishment and the inability to forgive oneself. Shame, however, is the individual's perception of being whole, deemed as faulty as an appliance. These powerful emotions are unhealthy as they render a person helpless and unable to improve his life.

LACK OF SELF-IDENTITY

Childhood with toxic parents has impacts on the child's emotional development, and one of them is the absence of personal identity. Such people may need an identity, goals and plans for the future, or personal philosophy in life. Negative messages conveyed to the target by toxic parents include criticism and withdrawal of support; the individual may have trouble defining themselves and, therefore, may fail to set personal objectives. It, therefore, results in, among others, feelings of confused self-identity, purposelessness, and inability to stand for themselves in various facets of their lives.

Relationship Challenges Stemming from Toxic Parenting

TRUST ISSUES

Trust is one of the elements that are hugely affected by toxic parenting when it comes to relationships in adulthood. Being raised in a context that entails promises, telling lies, or failing to meet the emotional requirements of other people disorients adults into not trusting people. Such people might always expect to be betrayed or believe that the expectations in a relationship will always be disappointed. Such mistrust results in long-standing stress and the impossibility of having significant relationships with others. This can be seen as jealousy, suspicion or the need to constantly check up on the partner, thereby putting pressure on the relationship.

DIFFICULTY SETTING BOUNDARIES

Some of the longer-term consequences are that those who were exposed to toxic parenting have difficulties in establishing and enforcing personal boundaries. They may have learned that their wants and needs are not as important as others; thus, they may be overly generous or perform excess or overwork to their detriment. In relationships, this leads to unhealthy selfishness, where they answer the needs of others while their own needs are poorly met; thus, post-ACT leads to resentment and burnout. Conversely, they would want to establish substantial barriers to avoid threats, which makes it hard to develop close relationships.

FEAR OF INTIMACY

This entry deals with intimacy and how it is a root fear for many grown-up children from toxic parents. These adults may have learned that closeness equals pain, manipulation or control over them into giving in to what is required. For this reason, they may avoid close relationships with other people so they do not get hurt. It may also work out as low emotional intimacy, preventing the expression of feelings or the constant breakup of relationships even before they reach a deeper level. Isolation from other people cements one's idea that they cannot be loved and cannot love in return, thus continuing the pattern.

DEPENDING ON OTHERS

It also produces codependency in mature relationships among adults as spoiling children turn into spoiled adult children. Codependency is a behavioral pattern that characterizes an individual who gets overly involved in their partner's life emotionally and focuses on getting validation from the partner. People may take on obligations for their partner's emotions and behaviors while neglecting themselves dramatically. This dynamic may bring out pathogenic patterns within relationships that may lead to enmeshment, where differentiation is a problem, and one's identity is held hostage to the other. Codependency is associated with a lack of independence, where people with the condition are likely to lack the ability to make decisions on their own because the consequences of decision-making scare them, such as the possibility of being abandoned or rejected by their loved ones.

REENACTMENT OF DYSFUNCTIONAL PATTERNS

Toxic parents negatively affect the normal development of a person, and they deprive them of essential skills, which have an impact towards toxic relational styles put in practice in adulthood. They might end up being involved in a relationship with personalities like the parent; these include being controlling, critical, or even emotionally distant. That is why this reenactment can bring some comfort, although it is somewhat pathological and produces toxic relationships only. It is critically important to identify them and change for recovery and to build new and better interactions.

Although the social stigma varies among pupils, Shamis has low self-esteem and needs validation from others. In turn, toxic parenting leads to low self-esteem and constant seeking for validation, which is not suitable for a person. In relationships, adults may require their partners to give them constant validation that we are helpful in society and that they need us. This overreliance on external validation can be highly problematic in a relationship as it places much pressure on the partners, who may feel ill-equipped to handle it. Also, based on the aspect of self-esteem, people who lack it will allow their partners to disrespect or mistreat them or remain in abusive relationships because they do not think they deserve better.

COMMUNICATION PROBLEMS

Social skills, especially verbal communication, are essential to healthy relationships. Nevertheless, toxic parenting affects people, and they may have problems with this. They could have grown up developing the ability not to express certain feelings or engage in arguments because of the household atmosphere. In adults, it leads to passive aggression, deficient functioning in expressing needs and wants, and temper tantrums when the parent's suppressed anger boils over. Lack of communication leads to hurt and anger, and the inability to solve petty differences leads to more negative effects in relations.

FEAR OF ABANDONMENT

Another issue often found is a person's fear of being abandoned. Some of those who were emotionally starved or abused by their parents are likely to be anxious that their partners will reject them. Such fear may result in bitter clinging and dependency or, on the other hand, counter dependent behavior to avoid the situation of getting abandoned. The level of fear implicitly transfers to anxiety and insecurity, which can prove catastrophic to any stable relationship because trust is hard to build, let alone be constant.

DIFFICULTY IN FORMING ATTACHMENTS

Thus, toxic parenting could alter the typical formation of healthy patterns of attachment. People in the adult groups can develop insecure models of the self and emotions, such as anxious or avoidant models. The fact that people with anxious attachment need closeness while at the same time feeling that there is no reciprocation from the partner creates clinginess and anxiety. The second type is the avoidantly attached people, who can usually have difficulties with building close and safe relationships as they prefer to avoid closeness to avoid pain. Both forms have severe implications for developing balanced mutual relationships in which each subject is an integral participant.

Such ordeals depict how pervasive toxic parenting is in precluding an individual from forging and maintaining relationships. These factors must be resolved with the help of self-awareness, therapy, and healthy interpersonal relationships to regain and establish good relationship patterns.

Breaking the Cycle: Avoiding Toxic Patterns in Your Own Parenting

Breaking free from the toxic patterns learned from your parentss can be challenging but is essential for creating a healthy, nurturing environment for your children. Here are strategies to help you avoid perpetuating toxic behaviors and foster a positive parenting approach:

SELF-AWARENESS AND REFLECTION

Recognize Your Triggers: This is often done about the activities that elicit negative responses or actions. How do these triggers fit with the childhood experiences you can relate to? If you can comprehend why, you are reacting the way you are, you will likely deal with it effectively.

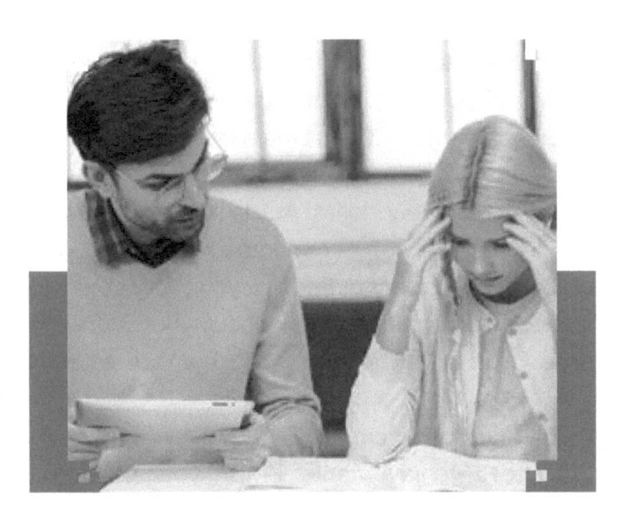

Acknowledge Your Emotions: Keep expressing your emotions genuinely and the impact you are experiencing as a parent. One can only act out the scripts of the self, and under repressed conditions, the behavioral scripts may turn into a semi-violent outburst in an attempt to express the suppressed feelings, or one can become quite passive-aggressive. A part of the self-care is to be able to allow yourself to feel and process these emotions.

POSITIVE COMMUNICATION

Active Listening: Take time to attend to what your children are saying. Make them understand that their thought process and feelings are being listened to. This creates rapport and fosters effective communication, which means there is likely to be something other than bitterness that arises from misunderstandings.

Express Yourself Clearly: Say one thing at the beginning of the sentence, then follow it with another thing- This can be in the style of 'I feel' or 'It is important that'. For example, use something like, "I get angry when the room is messy because I would want it clean," instead of saying, "You never tidy this room."

HEALTHY BOUNDARIES

Set Clear Expectations: Parents and children should clarify the rules and expectations early. To ensure young people appreciate these rules, use this approach because it helps them feel appreciated.

Respect Their Boundaries: Adults say 'stop', and so should your children – remember to respect your children's boundaries as much as you expect them to respect yours. Let them speak about what they want or need, using the theory of giving them self-esteem.

Positive Reinforcement

Celebrate Achievements: Praise your children's efforts and congratulate them even on their little achievements. Rewarding behavior increases the rate of occurrence of that particular behavior by making the person feel good about themselves.

CONSTRUCTIVE FEEDBACK:

- Acknowledge and transform the manner of feedback provision.
- Aim at the positive aspects that could be intervened and not the negative aspects that have been provided.
- Provide advice and assistance to enable them to be trained and evolve.

EMOTIONAL SUPPORT

Be Present: You should spend quality time with your children. Display concern in their activities and hear them out. Everyone gains something from being there and feels they are essential and part of something.

Validate Their Feelings: Always make your children feel that they are being accepted, even where they are coming from emotionally, though it may not make complete sense to you. Remind them that they have the right to feel the way they do. This validation builds up emotional strength and strengthens individuals to face adversity.

SELF-CARE AND PERSONAL GROWTH

Prioritize Self-Care: Take care of your health, both physical, emotional, and mental. While parenting can be challenging, self-care allows one to be healthy and patient enough to be a role model.

Seek Professional Help: If you have unresolved issues from your childhood, it will be helpful to turn to a therapist. If one has been through such experiences, one must seek the assistance of a professional so that the experiences can be dealt with and ways of handling them in healthier ways can be found.

MODEL HEALTHY RELATIONSHIPS

Demonstrate Respect: The roles include Demonstrating appropriate behavior to others. Children are watchers; thus, learning to respect other people in any of your relations passes the learning to the children.

Conflict Resolution: Dealing with conflict always in a civil manner. Explain ways in which people can handle conflict without aggression or persuasion. This gives your children excellent skills in solving disputes.

ENCOURAGING INDEPENDENCE

Empower Decision-Making: Let your children be independent and learn their lessons from the mistakes they make. This leads to independence and self-confidence, which must suit future employees.

Support Their Interests: Encourage your children in their education and hobbies that they have chosen, no matter how much they don't align with your preferences. Teasing out feedback that stops them from becoming their unique selves helps build healthy self-esteem.

CONSISTENT LOVE AND AFFECTION

Express Love Regularly: Show love and affection consistently. Physical touch, verbal affirmations, and quality time all convey love and security.

Create a Safe Environment: Make sure your home is a relatively secure environment for your children and they feel loved and wanted there. An environment that can be described as stable is essential for children's emotional growth.

Leaving toxic parenting behind is not an easy task; it necessitates purposeful actions, acknowledgement of the existing conditions, and the willingness of both parties involved. So, by incorporating these measures, you will be able to provide your children with the best conditions for their healthy development. Anyway, even the best parents can make mistakes; therefore, asking for advice and gradually improving is pretty normal. For this reason, your resolve to help end this cycle can go a long way in producing positive, healthy, and secure children.

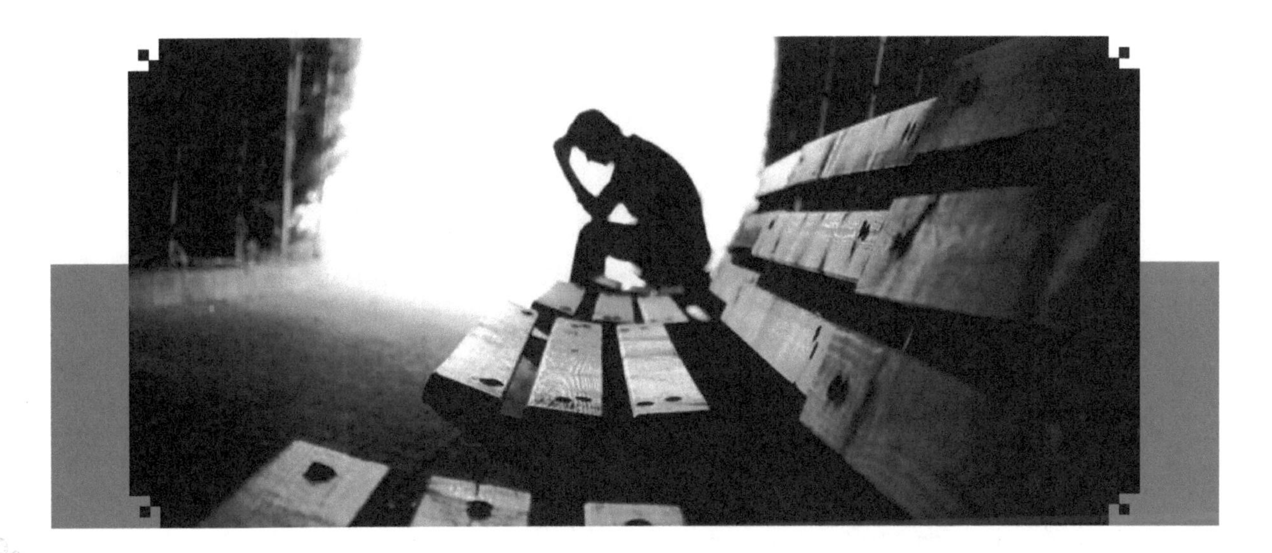

Chapter 4

Establishing Boundaries

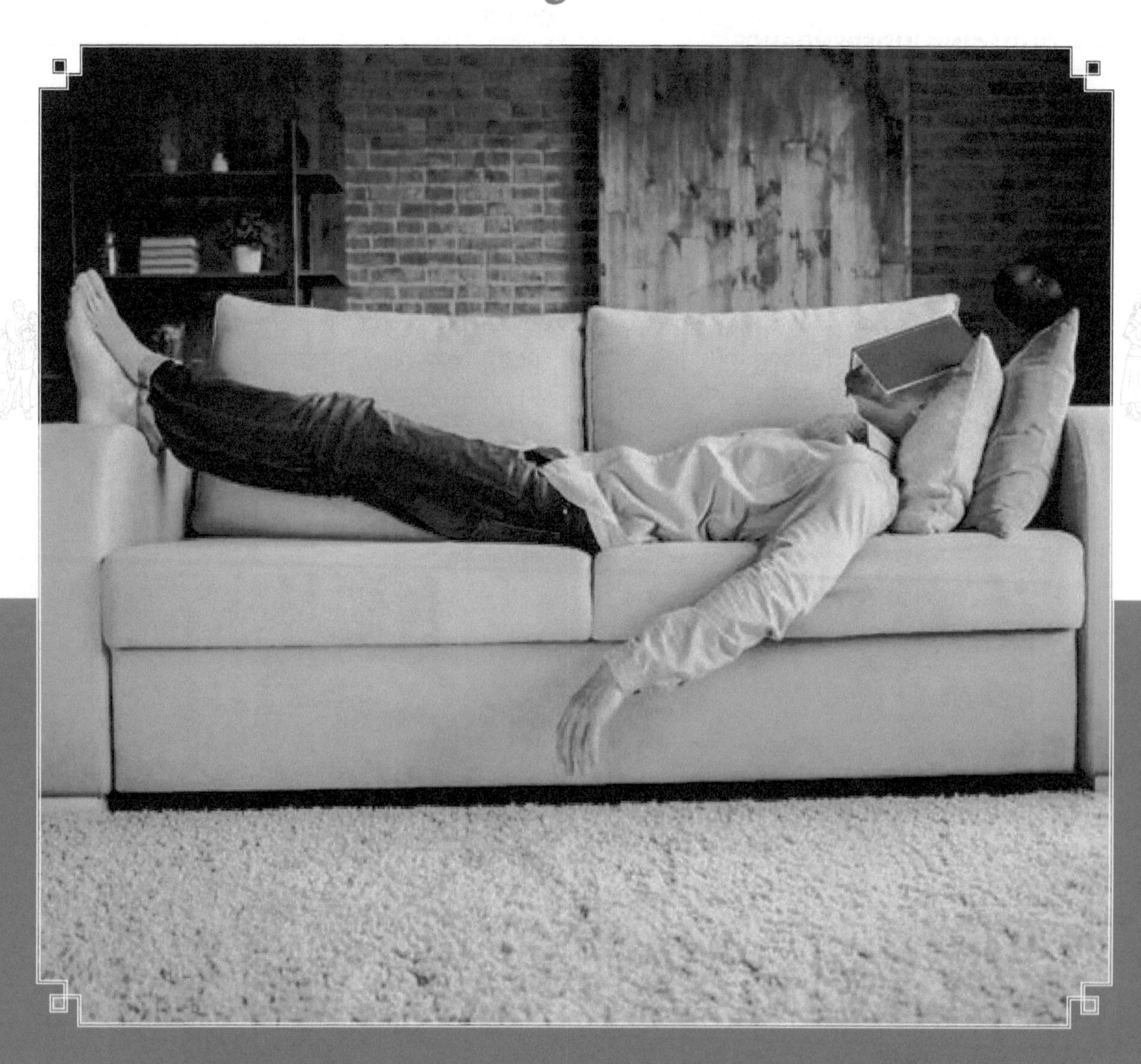

Some of the ways that are known to help are to set boundaries, which is a core part of emotional well-being and learning to be an individual, significantly if toxic parents raise one. It is understood that boundaries set the degree of tolerance one has for others and the standards that they are willing to allow others to set with them. It is very crucial and may, at the same time, be a strict regime for people who grew up in homes where boundaries were never crossed or nonexistent.

In other words, boundaries may be described as imaginary lines that help shield our spirit and psychological self. They assist in preserving their self-conception and self-esteem to remain intact and are necessary for proper interpersonal interactions.

The Importance of Setting Boundaries

By not respecting the child's boundaries, toxic parents end up corrupting the child's understanding of what is acceptable and what is not. For instance, the parent might violate the child's rights to privacy, disregard their emotions/needs, or set unrealistic demands. Such treatment is likely to make children feel they are nonentities and powerless; it also reduces married persons' ability to set healthy boundaries.

For that reason, it could be that you have a learning disability as an adult child of toxic parents and have developed unhealthy boundaries within yourself. This can present as trouble with identifying boundaries or saying 'no,' going out of one's way to meet other people's needs, or being oblivious to one's own needs and wants. These are some of the patterns one must detect to set up the proper boundary.

Below are some of the why it is wise to have boundaries:

Protecting Your Well-Being: Boundaries help a person create a limit that helps protect oneself and avoid harming one's emotions and mind. Avoid allowing people to treat you in a particular manner that you do not deserve because by having a set of DOs and DONTs, you are sure to be controlled while you control the environment around you. This protection is necessary so you do not suffer emotionally or get burnt out.

Fostering Healthy Relationships: Introduction The Consequences of transforming personal relationships into business-like ones are essential since they affect all spheres of people's lives. The integrity of interactions is a significant component of respect and fully satisfying partnerships in various spheres of people's lives. They assist in ensuring that your requirements and expectations are well understood, minimizing disputes. Of course, healthy boundaries help people express themselves and get respect from others, which is distinctive for any successful relationship.

Promoting Self-Respect: Specifically, the picture is an action that implies humility, while setting boundaries is a sign of respect towards oneself. It shows that you care for yourself and your needs and can't tolerate any inimical treatment to your health. This self-respect helps enhance a good image of oneself and improve one's self-worth.

Encouraging Personal Growth: These are important because boundaries generate the needed space for the growth of an individual. Thus, when setting limits, it is possible to put self-interest before the selfishness of others, devoting time to personal development and achievements. Such alters could be developed from this process, strengthening the person's identification.

Breaking the Cycle: For many, setting boundaries is a way to break free from unhealthy patterns established during childhood. By establishing clear limits, you challenge the toxic dynamics that may have been normalized in your upbringing. This act of defiance is crucial for healing and creating a healthier future.

How to Establish and Maintain Healthy Boundaries

Setting and especially practicing personal boundaries is conducive and essential for personal satisfaction and ensuring that all relationships with others are preferably healthy. Self-termination for adult child inmates is, for the most part, a devastating task but critical if they are going to be set free from toxic parents. Below is a detailed guideline to help you successfully set and maintain personal boundaries.

1. Self-Assessment: It is time to know your wants and no-wants.

Identify Your Boundaries: Start by including the probable self-requirements and self-impossibilities. Think about situations in which you get flustered, are demeaned or under pressure. These are feelings of where you have to draw the line, where you cannot let someone take advantage of you anymore. They may concern the physical proximity and separation, recognition of each other's rights to specific emotional states, time usage, or communication manner.

Recognize Your Patterns: Reflect on previous cases and the present relational patterns concerning boundaries. Do you often put up with others and do everything for them and yourself, too? Are you a person who has difficulties saying NO? Familiarizing yourself with these cycles can assist you in identifying when they are necessary and, potentially, why it was so difficult to establish them.

2. To make your boundaries clear and ensure you are the one setting them, you must be assertive.

USE "I" STATEMENTS:

- Avoid using accusatory language When enforcing your boundaries.
- Make sure you say things in a manner that you feel it.
- For instance, rewrite such comments as "I get annoyed every time you interrupt me" to "It bothers me when you interrupt me.

Be Specific and Direct: Spelling out what is required and expected in good detail. The use of certain generalities, which are unclear, leaves much room for ambiguity. For instance, rather than complain about, "I want more respect," say, "I want you to ask before using my items."

Remain Calm and Confident: Be assertive when practicing boundaries in a conversation with the perpetrators. It has enforcement or conflict consequences caused by the emotional reaction. Muster is the ability to stay calm and imposing when nastily answered by the other individual.

3. Set Realistic and Achievable Boundaries

Evaluate Feasibility: Ensure that the boundaries you set are realistic and achievable. Setting overly rigid or unrealistic boundaries can lead to frustration and conflict. Consider what is practical for you and the other party, and adjust your expectations as needed.

Balance Flexibility with Firmness: While being firm about your boundaries is essential, flexibility may be necessary depending on the context. For example, you might need to adapt your boundaries in a work setting compared to personal relationships. Strive for a balance that respects your needs while accommodating reasonable adjustments.

4. Enforce Boundaries Consistently
Follow Through: Consistency is critical to maintaining boundaries. If you set a boundary but do not enforce it, it can lead to confusion and disregard. Follow through with consequences if boundaries are violated, and remain steadfast in upholding them.

Reinforce Positive Behavior: When others respect your boundaries, acknowledge and appreciate their efforts. Positive reinforcement can encourage continued respect and foster a healthier relationship dynamic.

5. Manage Resistance and Guilt
Anticipate Pushback: Setting boundaries, especially with toxic individuals, may lead to resistance or adverse reactions. Prepare for this possibility and remain committed to your boundaries despite pushback. Understanding that resistance is a normal part of the process can help you stay focused and resilient.

Address Guilt: It's common to feel Guilt when setting boundaries, particularly if it conflicts with ingrained patterns from your upbringing. Remind yourself that setting boundaries is an act of self-care and self-respect. Prioritize your well-being and challenge any guilt by focusing on the positive impact of your boundaries.

6. If suffering from any mental health issues or stress, get help for themselves and remain patient with their healing.

Consider Professional Guidance: If setting or maintaining boundaries proves difficult, the best action plan is to approach a therapist or a counsellor. It is suggested that professional advice be sought on enforcing boundaries and coping with any arising emotional issues.

Practice Self-Care: It is essential to note that personal boundaries are very much related to self-care. Activities that allow you to step back from your working life can maintain your disciplinary boundaries. Practical activities beneficial in strengthening tough-mindedness's psychological processes include self-care, relaxation, meditation, and hobbies.

Dealing with Resistance and Guilt

The most common difficulty associated with resistance is Guilt concerning the boundary process; this tends to be a significant problem for toxic parent survivors. It is essential to manage these sensations to keep the boundaries healthy and safe for the survivor. Here's a guide to help you address resistance and Guilt effectively: Here's a guide to help you address resistance and Guilt effectively:

1. Understanding Resistance
Recognize the Sources of Resistance: There are internal and external sources of resistance, such as the internal self and people you affect through your boundaries. Some employees might not wish to change because they are comfortable with the previous methods, or they derive some form of satisfaction from protracted conflicts at the workplace. Internal barriers can also be attributed to such challenges as conflict in dealing with aggressors and perceived effects on relational dynamics.

Anticipate and Prepare for Pushback: Be ready for the fact that to set boundaries is possibly to meet some opposition or discomfort, especially with people who aren't used to your rules. One should prepare for the promotion of adverse reactions since it can help you stick to your position and act based on it.

2. Strategies for Managing Resistance

Stay Firm and Consistent: As can be seen, consistency is essential when handling resistance. It is necessary to stay guarded by the rules once they have been set and not budge when people resist. Regular use of the regulations enforces them to ensure clients understand that some rules are unchangeable.

Communicate Clearly and Calmly:

- When dealing with resistance, stay focused on setting boundaries and do so composedly.
- Do not argue, and do not become angry.
- Remind your partner about your needs simply and clearly, explaining how the boundary benefits both of you.

Set Consequences if Necessary: Thus, if necessary, guidelines can be established for reprimand in the case of continued breaches of the boundaries. For instance, if a person treats your time with disdain, you would not make yourself available to that individual. Ensure the consequence you derive elicits equity and has a clear correlation with the established boundary.

Acknowledge and Validate Their Feelings: There might be value in stating clearly the other person's feelings about the boundary. Confirming their feelings does not necessarily mean that you must bypass your barrier more, which is nonetheless considerate and may help defuse the situation. For example, "I realize that this may not sit well with you, but this is something that I must do for myself."

3. Addressing Guilt

Understand the Source of Guilt: A feeling of Guilt recoils from the goal of people's disappointment or disturbance in a relationship. It can also originate from people-pleasing behavior or feeling like you must meet a duty. It is essential to differentiate the core of your Guilt so that you can try to solve it correctly.

Reframe Your Perspective: Change your perspective about boundaries from selfish acts to protective measures for one's well-being. This calms your conscience each time you set boundaries, and it helps you understand that it is healthy to set these boundaries for the sake of your well-being and healthier relationships. These guidelines regulate relations and help maintain an appropriate working and free time ratio to avoid exhaustion.

Challenge Negative Self-Talk: Judgement, a kind of negative self-talk or self-criticism, can intensify Guilt. Overcome such thoughts with the help of the positive consequences of boundaries and appreciation of oneself. You can also remind yourself that it is healthy and essential to set your limits and know your limitations.

Practice Self-Compassion: Take it easy with yourself as you try to assert yourself in this process. Accept the fact that you have got the hormones of Guilt running, but understand that it's normal and you are using your best judgement. Self-compassion entails recognizing one's efforts and knowing that one should be given equal regard as any other human being.

Seek Support and Validation: It's good to share with a mental health professional or a counsellor or attend a support group offering guidance and validation.

Support from others who understand the challenges of setting boundaries can help you navigate feelings of Guilt and reinforce your commitment to maintaining healthy limits.

4. Self-Care and Reflection
Engage in Self-Care: Engaging in behaviors that enable you to reduce stress and effectively maintain a healthy emotional balance is essential. It is also encouraging to practice quitting toxic habits and engaging in more productive things such as exercising, doing hobbies and practicing mindfulness to build resilience in handling resistance and Guilt.

Reflect on Your Progress: As a self-reflection, frequently contemplate your interactions with boundaries, dealing with resistance and Guilt included. Determine the outcomes of the implementation of specific approaches to performance and identify areas where changes may be appropriate. It can also make you feel more confident about setting appropriate boundaries for yourself.

5. Moving Forward
Embrace the Learning Process: Understanding and managing resistance and Guilt is ongoing. Please take it as constructive criticism and use it as a stepping stone to personal growth and having a better relationship. All the measures that are taken in the process of building and enforcing the boundaries contribute to the development of personal protection mechanisms.

Balanced and fulfilling life.
An even more important practice is knowing how to handle resistance and Guilt when putting into operation and enforcing boundaries. If you know how to handle sources of resistance, cope with them efficiently, address the issues of Guilt with self-compassion, and incorporate self-care strategies. You will be prepared to face this process effectively. As already mentioned, this is an effective practice in protecting your emotional health and self-development and serves as a basis for forming more civilized and proper behavior between people.

Practical Exercises for Boundary Setting

Boundaries are an aspect of life that can be set and changed from time to time, and thus, the understanding of boundary setting is correct. Here are some practical exercises designed to help you build confidence and effectiveness in setting and maintaining boundaries: Here are some practical exercises designed to help you build confidence and effectiveness in setting and keeping boundaries:

1. Reflective Journaling
Objective: Increase self-awareness about your boundaries and identify areas needing improvement.

HOW TO DO IT:
Daily Reflection: At the end of each day, write about any situations where your boundaries were tested or violated. Note how you responded and how you felt.

Identify Patterns: Look for recurring themes or patterns in your reflections. Are there specific people or situations that frequently challenge your boundaries?

Clarify Needs: Write about what you need in these situations to feel respected and safe. Be specific about the boundaries you want to set.

EXAMPLE JOURNAL PROMPTS:
"Today, I felt uncomfortable when [specific situation]. I wish I had set a boundary by [desired response]."
"I often struggle with boundaries when [describe situation]. What could I do differently?"

2. Boundary Role-Playing

Objective: Practice asserting boundaries in a controlled environment to build confidence.

HOW TO DO IT:

Select Scenarios: Choose common scenarios where you struggle with boundaries. These could be related to work, family, or social situations.

Partner Role-Play: With a trusted friend or therapist, role-play these scenarios. Take turns practicing how you would assert your boundaries.

Receive Feedback: After each role-play, discuss what felt comfortable and what could be improved. Use this feedback to refine your approach.

EXAMPLE SCENARIOS:

A coworker continually interrupts you during meetings.

A family member frequently asks for help at inconvenient times.

3. Visualization Exercise

Objective: Strengthen your mental resilience and prepare for boundary-setting in real situations.

HOW TO DO IT:

Find a Quiet Space: Sit in a quiet space where you can relax and focus.

Visualize a Scenario: Imagine a specific situation where you must set a boundary. Visualize yourself responding assertively and calmly.

Experience the Outcome: Picture the positive outcome of your boundary-setting, such as feeling empowered or the other person respecting your limits.

Repeat: Practice this visualization exercise regularly to reinforce your confidence and readiness.

Visualization Example:

"Imagine your friend is asking for a favor you can't accommodate. Visualize yourself saying, 'I'm unable to help with this request. I need to focus on my tasks right now.' See the friend's reaction and your feelings of relief and confidence."

4. Boundary Affirmations

Objective: Reinforce your self-worth and commitment to setting boundaries.

HOW TO DO IT:

Create Affirmations: Develop positive affirmations reinforcing your right to set and maintain boundaries. Focus on your worth and the importance of self-respect.

Daily Repetition: Repeat these affirmations in the morning or before challenging situations. Say them out loud or write them down.

EXAMPLE AFFIRMATIONS:

"I have the right to set boundaries that protect my well-being."

"My needs and feelings are valid, and I deserve respect."

5. Boundary-Setting Practice with "I" Statements

Objective: Develop practical communication skills for asserting boundaries.

HOW TO DO IT:

Identify Boundary Needs: List situations where you must set boundaries using "I" statements.

Draft Statements: Write clear, assertive "I" statements that express your needs and limits. Ensure they are direct and non-accusatory.

EXAMPLE STATEMENTS:

"I need time to recharge after work. Please do not call me during this time unless it's an emergency."
"I feel uncomfortable when you interrupt me during meetings. I need to finish my thoughts before responding."

6. Boundary Checklist
Objective: Ensure that your boundaries are well-defined and effectively communicated.

HOW TO DO IT:

Create a Checklist: Develop a checklist of essential boundary-setting components, including clarity, assertiveness, consistency, and follow-through.
Evaluate Your Boundaries: Regularly review and evaluate your boundaries against this checklist to ensure they are effectively set and maintained.

CHECKLIST COMPONENTS:

Clarity: Are your boundaries clear and specific?
Assertiveness: Are you expressing your boundaries confidently and respectfully?

Consistency: Are you consistently enforcing your boundaries?
Follow-Through: Are there appropriate consequences for boundary violations?

7. SELF-CARE PLANNING

Objective: Integrate boundary-setting into your self-care routine to ensure boundaries are honored.

HOW TO DO IT:

Identify Self-Care Needs: List activities and practices that support your well-being, such as relaxation, hobbies, or personal time.

Integrate Boundaries: Ensure your self-care needs are respected by setting boundaries around these activities. Communicate your needs to others and prioritize self-care.

SELF-CARE EXAMPLES:

"I need uninterrupted time each day for exercise and relaxation. Please respect this time and avoid scheduling other activities during it."

"I will not check work emails after 7 PM to ensure I have time to unwind."

Practical exercises for boundary setting can significantly enhance your ability to establish and maintain healthy limits. By engaging in reflective journaling, role-playing, visualization, affirmations, practicing "I" statements, using a boundary checklist, and planning for self-care, you can build confidence and resilience in setting boundaries. These exercises help you assert your needs effectively and contribute to your overall emotional well-being and healthier relationships.

Case Studies: Success Stories in Boundary Setting

Hearing about real-life success stories can be incredibly inspiring and provide practical insights into how boundary setting can transform relationships and personal well-being. Here are several case studies illustrating how individuals successfully established and maintained boundaries:

Case Study 1: Emily and Her Overbearing Mother
Background: Emily, a 32-year-old graphic designer, had always felt overwhelmed by her mother's constant involvement. Her mother would drop by unannounced, call multiple times daily, and offer unsolicited advice about every aspect of Emily's life.

Challenge: Emily felt suffocated and lacked personal space but feared hurting her mother's feelings if she set boundaries.

Action Taken: Emily decided to have an open and honest conversation with her mother. She expressed her need for personal space and privacy, emphasizing that she loved her mother but needed some boundaries to maintain her mental health.

Implemented Boundaries: Emily asked her mother to call before visiting and to limit phone calls to once a day unless it was an emergency.

Follow-Through: When her mother initially resisted and continued her old patterns, Emily firmly reminded her of their agreement and held her ground.

Outcome: Over time, her mother began to respect Emily's boundaries. Their relationship improved as Emily felt less stressed and more in control of her life. Her mother also learned to appreciate and respect Emily's need for independence.

Key Takeaway: Honest communication and consistent follow-through can help establish and maintain boundaries, even with close family members.

Case Study 2: James and His Demanding Boss
Background: James, a 45-year-old marketing manager, had a boss who frequently demanded overtime and weekend work without prior notice. This left James with little time for his family and personal life.

Challenge: James felt pressured to comply with his boss's demands to avoid conflict or appearing uncommitted to his job.

Action Taken: After experiencing burnout, James set boundaries to protect his work-life balance. He scheduled a meeting with his boss to discuss the issue.

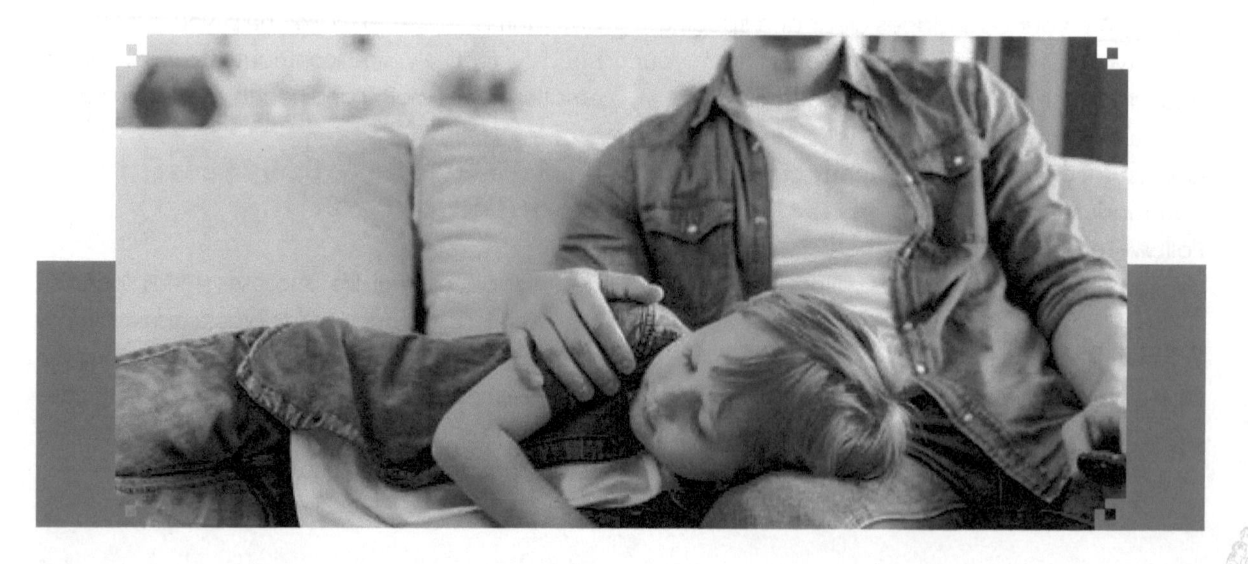

Implemented Boundaries: James communicated his willingness to work hard during business hours but expressed that he needed evenings and weekends for family time. He proposed a system for urgent tasks that respected his off-hours.

Follow-Through: When his boss made unreasonable requests outside of agreed hours, James reminded him of their conversation and suggested rescheduling the tasks for the next business day.

Outcome: James's boss initially struggled with the change but eventually adapted. James found a significant improvement in his work-life balance, which enhanced his productivity and job satisfaction. His boss also started respecting other employees' boundaries, improving workplace morale.

Key Takeaway: Professional boundaries can be set through clear communication and practical solutions, leading to better work-life balance and improved job performance.

Case Study 3: Rachel and Her Friend Group

Background: Rachel, a 28-year-old teacher, had friends who often pressured her to join social events even when she needed time to rest and recharge. She felt guilty saying no and usually ended up feeling exhausted and resentful.

Challenge: Rachel struggled with asserting her needs for fear of being seen as unsociable or losing her friends.

Action Taken: Rachel decided to communicate her needs openly with her friends. She explained that she valued their friendship but also needed time to maintain her energy and well-being.

Implemented Boundaries: Rachel set a boundary of limiting social outings to once or twice a week and being transparent about her availability.

Follow-Through: When friends pressured her beyond her limits, she politely but firmly declined, reinforcing her boundaries.

Outcome: Rachel's friends initially had difficulty adjusting but eventually understood and respected her needs. Rachel found that her friendships grew more assertive as her friends appreciated her honesty, and she could enjoy social events without feeling overwhelmed.

Key Takeaway: Setting boundaries in social relationships can enhance the quality of interactions and ensure personal well-being.

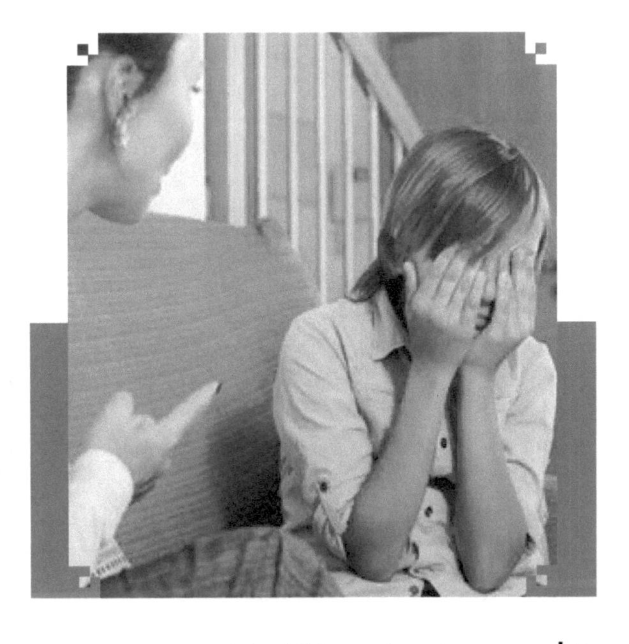

Case Study 4: Tom and His Workaholic Tendencies

Background: Tom, a 38-year-old software engineer, tended to overcommit to work on projects, often working late into the night and on weekends. This behavior strained his relationship with his partner and affected his health.

Challenge: Tom felt compelled to prove his dedication to his job but realized he was sacrificing his personal life and well-being.

Action Taken: Tom decided to set clear boundaries between his work and personal life. He communicated his new working hours with his team and committed to sticking to them.

Implemented Boundaries: Tom set a rule to stop working by 6 PM and not to work on weekends unless necessary.

Follow-Through: He used time management tools to priorities tasks and avoid overcommitment. When tempted to work late, he reminded himself of his commitment to his health and relationship.

Outcome: Tom's productivity during work hours improved, and he experienced less stress. His relationship with his partner strengthened as they spent more quality time together. Tom also felt healthier and more energized.

Key Takeaway: Personal boundaries regarding work can prevent burnout and improve overall life satisfaction.

These case studies illustrate that setting and maintaining boundaries, although challenging at first, can significantly improve personal well-being, relationships, and professional life. The key lies in clear communication, consistent follow-through, and being firm yet respectful in enforcing boundaries. Each success story highlights that with determination and practice, it is possible to create a healthier, more balanced life by establishing boundaries.

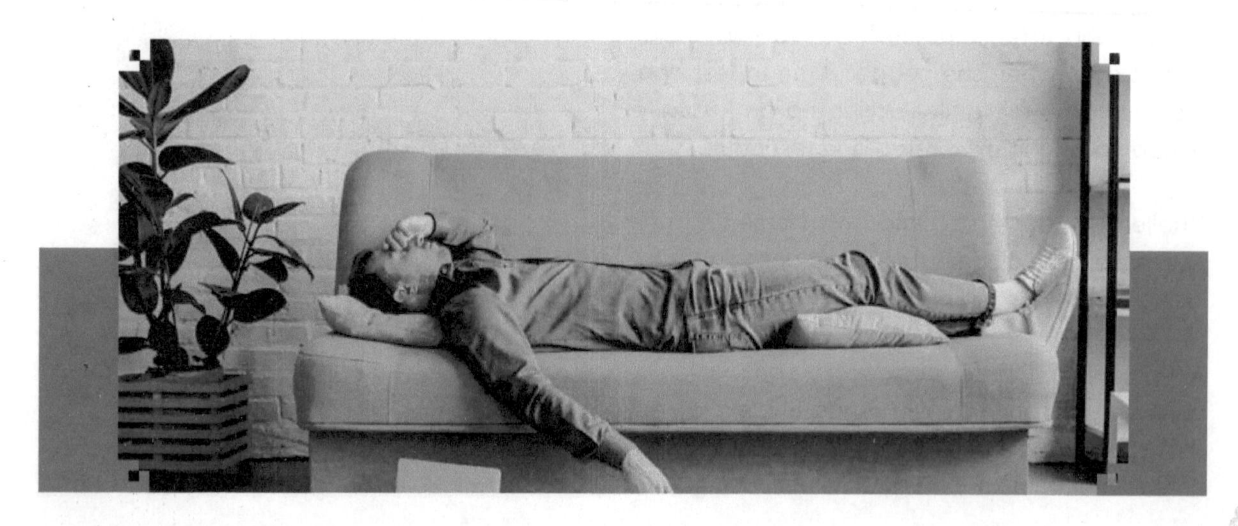

Chapter 5

Reclaiming Your Emotional Autonomy

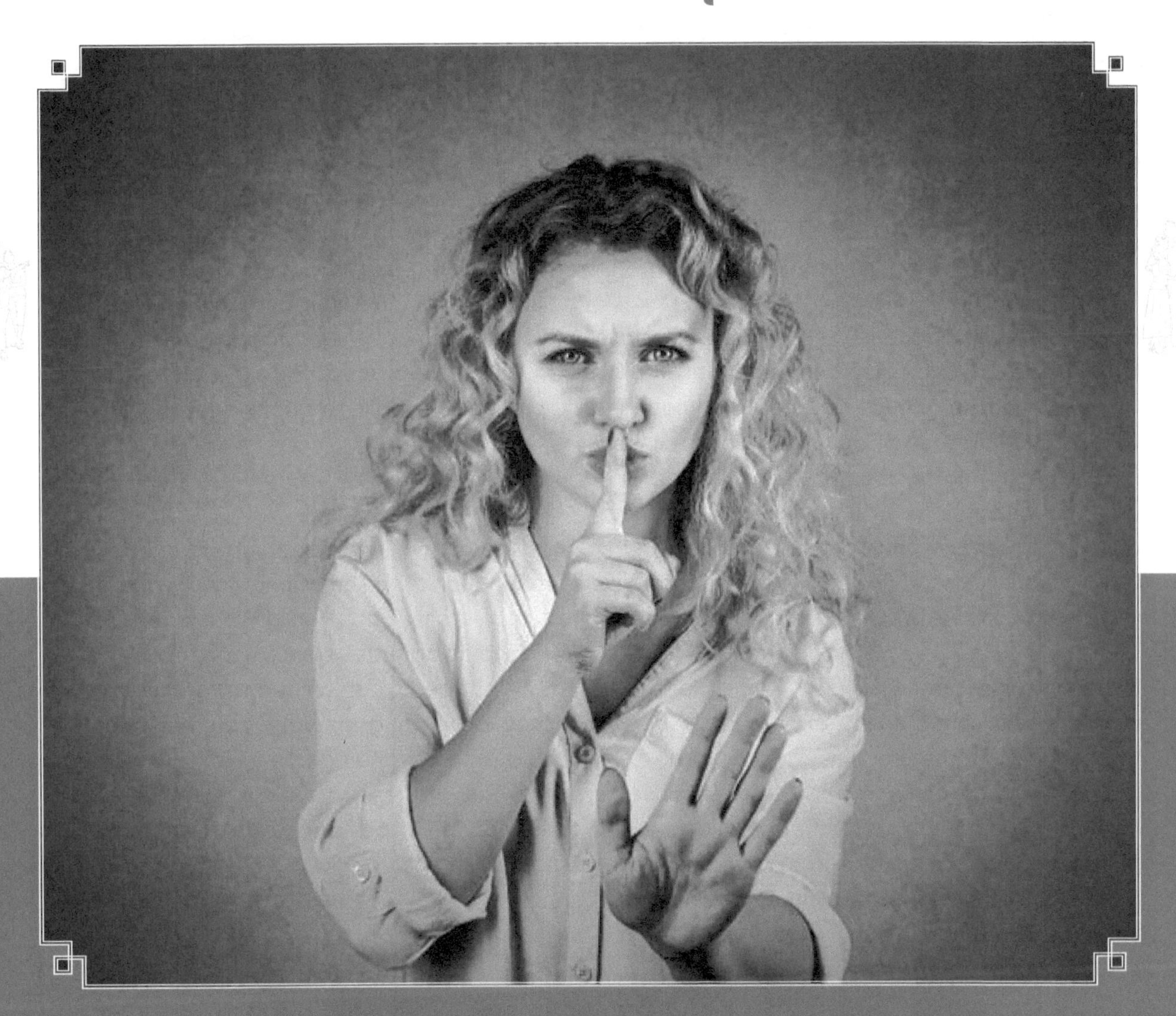

During the process of self-recovery from the expression of toxic parents, the most liberating thing you can do is to regain your right to feel. Emotional self-sufficiency refers to a person's capacity to regulate and control their feelings without interference from other people. For those growing up in toxic parent households, this entails having to undo the unhealthy and unhealthy actions of the parents and seek to embrace adulthood and wholesome boundaries, as well as having to find one's genuine emotional self. This section will provide the tools necessary to regain emotional freedom, including comprehensive lists of actions and strategies for creating the awareness, empathy, and strength required for a healthy life. Hence, with emotional independence as a guide, one can lead a more truthful, healthy, and happy existence.

Understanding Emotional Autonomy

Emotional self-reliance is the first step towards liberty and psychological wellness. It entails being able to experience and control emotions without the influence of other people's feelings. Parents toxic mothers or fathers become an essential principle for adult children when they attempt to remain emotionally detached from those who influenced not only their reaction on the emotional level but also personality inputs.

Emotional self-sufficiency means it is possible to feel emotions and control them simultaneously, being independent of other people's opinions or help. It means having the ability to pinpoint how one feels, know why one feels this or that, as well as how to put this into words without harming oneself or other people. Emotional self-reliance means owning up to your emotions rather than waiting for external stimuli or syncing with other people's feelings.

In childhood, the individuals were exposed to a toxic environment, and therefore, demonstrating emotional autonomy can be difficult. Thus, poisonous parents develop a pattern of behavior in which children's feelings are negated, controlled, or disregarded. Consequently, adult children are left reeling from numerous issues, such as low self-esteem, anxiety and deficits in their ability to trust their own emotions. This means regaining control of one's feelings to overcome such cycles and create a new and healthier way of experiencing feelings.

Steps to Reclaiming Your Emotional Independence

Getting over the effects of toxic parenting, therefore, requires that you first of all ensure that you get your emotional freedom back. It includes re-establishing the self, personal identity, the ability to draw the line, and self-nurture. Here are some critical steps to guide you in this transformative process: Here are some essential steps to guide you in this transformative process:

1. RECOGNIZE AND ACKNOWLEDGE YOUR EMOTIONAL PATTERNS

The first level of emotional individuation is the identification of the emotional scripts and stimuli resulting from one's childhood socialization. Read your parents' dance and contemplate how it shaped your emotional processes and strategies. Writing a diary can be helpful in such a process; one can define typical patterns in feelings and responses. It is indeed essential to identify such patterns to be free from toxic emotional attachment.

2. ESTABLISH CLEAR BOUNDARIES

Boundaries are a necessity for the recovery of one's emotionally independent state. Culturally imposed and prescribed standards of behaviors towards the opposite sex are the construct referred to as boundaries, which, when learnt, state what is allowed and prohibited in relationships and protect your emotional health. To begin with, one should define the need for boundaries, whether it is family members, friends, or work colleagues. Life situations often require people to set limits and explain this to others by being firm about them and ready to act them out. It is critical to note that boundaries are not tools for penalizing other people but for protecting oneself's well-being.

3. DEVELOP A STRONG SENSE OF SELF

Self-development is the process of developing self-acceptance, self-realization, and self-identity. Participate in interventions that can help one to understand oneself better: therapy, self-help, introspection, etc. Be decisive and discover what really and truly matters to you, then make choices in the light of that. In this way, asserting a positive self-image gives you more space for regulating your emotions and becoming more immune to others' opinions.

4. BUILD A SUPPORTIVE NETWORK

Although emotional independence implies that one must depend on oneself emotionally, having people to count on is always helpful. To solve this problem, one needs to strive to meet positive people who can encourage them and, at the same time, keep their boundaries. Be with people who support you and do not mind having you cry in front of them whenever you feel like it. Family and friends may have a different approach to helping, which can also strengthen the perception of being independent of one's emotions.

5. LEARN AND PRACTICE HEALTHY COPING STRATEGIES

Coping with emotional stress and minor disabilities to avoid reliance on others has to do with having suitable and healthy response mechanisms. Try activities like mindfulness, meditation, exercises or art to define the best ways to ease stress. Test different strategies to understand what is more effective in coping with stress and dealing with feelings. By adopting these approaches into your daily schedule and processes, you increase your coping capacity and stand a better chance of facing your emotions on your terms.

6. SET AND PURSUE PERSONAL GOALS

Having personal objectives and planning to achieve them is an effective means of supporting one's psychological emancipation. This means they must be acknowledged because they offer direction and purpose different from goals that target personal development and achievements. Find out which spheres of life one or multiple would like to change or improve and define corresponding strategies and tactics. It is essential to especially commemorate achievements, no matter how minor, as it makes the individual feel that they are in control and have some sense of value.

7. SEEK PROFESSIONAL SUPPORT IF NEEDED

Taking back one's emotions is not easy, which means that when people put themselves up for therapy, they are strong. It is recommended to seek help from a therapist or counsellor who will offer assistance, resources, and advice concerning your process. Such support is most needed in resolving emotional problems rooted in the individual and learning more valuable responses to stress. If dealing with such a task is a problem, do not be bold in your assistance.

Techniques for Self-Validation and Self-Care

Self-approval and self-feeding processes are significant activities that are helpful in maintaining a stable emotional status and non-dependence. It includes acknowledging and valuing oneself and one's needs besides undertaking the process of caring for oneself. Here are some effective techniques for incorporating self-validation and self-care into your life: Here are some practical methods for incorporating self-validation and self-care into your life:

1. PRACTICE SELF-COMPASSION

This is where people are kind and understanding towards themselves, just like they are to their friends. When things go wrong or if you make a mistake, allow yourself to feel whatever comes up without strangulation. This message should help the person remember that other people also have problems and Nobody is perfect. Techniques for practicing self-compassion include: Techniques for practicing self-compassion include:

Self-Talk: Avoid self-criticizing, insulting and hostile self-talk when talking to yourself. It is essential to work on positive self-talk instead of focusing on negative thinking.

Mindfulness: Practice mindfulness so that you can be aware of your thoughts and feelings but do not have to own them.

Self-Soothing: Employ calming functions, which include bathing with hot water, listening to your favorite music or engaging in a loved activity.

2. SET PERSONAL BOUNDARIES

Boundaries are essential as they help people know how far they can go and what they cannot do. People have boundaries that protect them and their feelings and make sure people around them meet their needs.

Techniques for setting boundaries include:

Identifying Limits: Define what is acceptable to you in different areas of your life: business, family, friends, and leisure.

Communicating Clearly: Be assertive when communicating your limitation to others; this means you have to avoid using phrases like 'you always' or 'you never,' but instead use words like 'I feel' or 'I need.'

Enforcing Boundaries: Admirably, consistently implement the set rules and always stand ready to give the much-needed corrective measures when needed.

3. ENGAGE IN REGULAR SELF-REFLECTION

It is also essential in the aspect of self-reflection to be able to discern one's needs, future aspirations, and emotions. First, analyze the patterns, get insight into your feelings, and then manage these emotions through the self-care plan. Techniques for self-reflection include:

Journaling: You ought to write frequently about your thoughts, feelings, and experiences. This practice can help clarify your emotions and identify patterns.

Meditation: It calms the mind and will allow you to explore your feelings and make personal discoveries about your internal world.

Feedback: Consider what others have shared and what you have learned regarding your self-care strategies.

4. DEVELOP A SELF-CARE ROUTINE

Creating a self-care routine ensures you regularly engage in activities promoting your well-being. Techniques for developing a self-care routine include:

Daily Practices: Incorporate small self-care activities into your daily schedule, such as taking breaks, practicing gratitude, or engaging in physical activity.

Weekly Rituals: Set aside time each week for self-care activities that recharge you, such as spending time with loved ones, pursuing hobbies, or practicing relaxation techniques.

Self-Care Plan: Develop a personalized self-care plan that includes activities you enjoy and that address your specific needs.

5. CULTIVATE POSITIVE SELF-AFFIRMATIONS

Self-affirmations help in the process of positive imaging and assist in the enhancement of self-esteem. Techniques for using self-affirmations include: Techniques for using self-affirmations include:

Daily Affirmations: Before going to sleep, close your eyes and silently say positive messages you want to hear from others, like "You are loved" or "You are strong.

Visual Reminders: Put the affirmations out where they can be seen daily, near the mirror or the desk, for instance, to be constantly in touch with the positive qualities.

Affirmation Practice: Building upon it by incorporating affirmations into your meditations or reflections is possible.

6. PRIORITIZE PHYSICAL HEALTH

Physical health is closely linked to emotional well-being. Taking care of your body supports overall self-care. Techniques for prioritizing physical health include:

Balanced Diet: Eat a nutritious diet that supports physical and mental health.

Regular Exercise: Engage in regular physical activity, such as walking, yoga, or strength training, to boost your mood and energy levels.

Adequate Rest: Sleep enough to support your physical and emotional recovery.

7. SEEK AND ACCEPT SUPPORT

While self-validation and self-care involve self-reliance, seeking and accepting support from others can enhance your well-being. Techniques for seeking and receiving support include:

Building Connections: Form friendships with good-natured people who embrace your decision and are patient, encouraging, and careful with your feelings.

Therapy or Counseling: One may want to ask for help from a healthcare professional to define and combat responses to emotional difficulties.

Support Groups: Get involved with other people going through similar situations where you can get that understanding and reassurance from other people.

8. ENGAGE IN JOYFUL ACTIVITIES

The assumption that self-care can include activities that make people happy and satisfied with their lives is accurate.

Techniques for engaging in joyful activities include:
Hobbies: Engage yourself in things that you think are fun, for instance, painting, gardening, reading or any other activity that would make you happy.

Creativity: Find hobbies that allow you to be creative, whether it is writing, sewing, film, or music, and find a little satisfaction in the completion of tasks.

Social Time: Hanging out with people that make you more enthusiastic about life and who you enjoy being around.

Older people particularly can well understand that applying these techniques in everyday practice will help them create a program that provides self-validation and contributes to improving one's quality of life. Self-care, though, is a progressive process. In this case, it becomes essential to monitor the effectiveness of such practices routinely and make changes as they may be needed.

Building Emotional Intelligence

Emotional intelligence can be defined as the capacity to perceive, appraise, and express emotions and manage them in oneself, as well as to affect the emotional climate of others. It is vital to note that emotional intelligence improves your social plans, personality, and health. Here are critical strategies for building emotional intelligence. Here are key strategies for building emotional intelligence:

1. SELF-AWARENESS

Self-awareness is the foundation of emotional intelligence. It involves recognizing your emotions, understanding their impact, and knowing your strengths and weaknesses.

Keep a Journal: Feel free to jot down how you feel and what you go through each day. Meditate on how you think and how these feelings affect your thoughts and actions.

Identify Triggers: Watch out for triggers; these are conditions or instances that elicit extreme feelings of passion. Knowing them allows you to avoid getting worked up over them or respond better when upset.

Seek Feedback: Request people's opinions on how they perceive your emotional reactions from friends, relatives or coworkers so that you can know how to handle them.

2. SELF-REGULATION

Self-regulation is the ability to control one's responses to the emotions that one experiences. Instead of giving an instant emotional response, it assists in formulating a constructive action plan.

Practice Mindfulness: To manage stress, practice relaxation procedures, meditation, or deeper breathing.

Develop Coping Strategies: Learn specific ways to relax and rehearse them to do them when you become stressed, such as taking a walk, practicing relaxation exercises, or positive self-talk.

Set Emotional Goals: Make concrete deadlines for regulating your emotions, including what kind you would like to work on today or this week, for instance, patience or impulsive behavior, and then measure yourself in a week or a month.

3. MOTIVATION

Intrinsic motivation is the drive to achieve goals for personal satisfaction and growth. It involves setting and pursuing meaningful goals and maintaining a positive attitude despite setbacks.

Set Personal Goals: Ensure you have personal goals that you will need to work towards, including choosing goals you are interested in and goals that uphold some of your personable values. It was advised to divide them into chunks to avoid demotivation and burnout.

Celebrate Achievements: There is nothing wrong with taking time and congratulating yourself for the work that you have achieved. This helps enhance a positive attitude toward the goal and thus ensures that the individual does not give up easily.

4. EMPATHY

Empathy is communication in which one tries to feel what the other person is feeling. It encompasses listening with the spirit and purpose of counselling, which involves the expression of sympathy and empathy towards the listener.

Listen Actively: Practice active listening by respecting the other person's turn to speak, thinking about the emotions they might be experiencing, and acknowledging those emotions.

Practice Perspective-Taking: Understanding how other people perceive matters is very important. This makes it easier for you to comprehend how they commonly feel and their reaction.

Respond with Empathy: In your communication approach, grant sympathy and encouragement. Applaud others' efforts, and appear supportive at the end of the conversation if you feel that they need your help.

5. SOCIAL SKILLS

Practical social skills are essential for building and maintaining healthy relationships. They involve communication, conflict resolution, and collaboration.

Improve Communication: That's why one needs to focus on improving communication skills, specifically by practicing cuteness and assertiveness. If you want to address your needs and feelings and avoid blaming others, use "I" statements.

Develop Conflict Resolution Skills: Acquire and apply skills used when addressing disputes, for example, searching and finding consensus, bargaining for a solution, and handling conflicts nonviolently.

6. SELF-CARE AND RESILIENCE

One should also appreciate personal health and well-being as products of emotional intelligence. These include maintenance of one's health and ability to deal with arising issues.

Prioritize Self-Care: Exercise, eat healthily and take time off to relax. All these are self-care measures that every person should take to ensure they remain spiritually and physically fit.

Build Resilience: We must strengthen the 'coping' factor of stress by adopting positivity and embracing the change of being unable to avoid stressors and learning to grow from them.

7. CONTINUOUS LEARNING

Emotional intelligence is a lifelong journey. Continuously seek opportunities for learning and growth to enhance your emotional skills.

Read and Learn: Explore books, articles, and courses on emotional intelligence and related topics. Stay updated on new strategies and insights.

Reflect and Adapt: Regularly reflect on your emotional experiences and progress. Adjust the tactics you used to enhance your emotional quotient as you go through various stages.

Practice and Apply: Always practice what you are taught in a real-life environment. Another is the repeated use of knowledge that supports the implementation of emotional intelligence in clients' everyday lives.

Thus, nurturing these elements of emotional intelligence directly contributes to your capacity to embrace and regulate emotions, sustain interpersonal relationships, and cope with life's stressors. So, it is essential to know that emotional intelligence is a skill that constantly evolves with practice and effort.

Mindfulness Practices for Emotional Health

Mindfulness is being present and fully engaged in the current moment without judgment. It has been shown to improve emotional health by reducing stress, enhancing self-awareness, and fostering greater well-being. Here are several mindfulness practices to support emotional health:

1. MINDFUL BREATHING

Mindful breathing involves awareness of breath to bring the individual's attention to the current moment. Stress is something that is disliked by many, and this can assist in the diminishing of stress.

Essential Breathing Exercise: Find or get a comfortable position or seating. Sit comfortably, close your eyes softly, and focus on the breath. Breathe through your nose while counting to five; feel your stomach expand; breathe out through your mouth, counting to five as your stomach contracts. Concentrate on the feeling of cold air entering your body through the nose and 'cool' air coming out of it. This should be done for 5-10 minutes daily.

Counting Breaths: To extend the focus, count your breaths from one to two and repeat this process continuously. Take a deep breath and say the first name aloud, counting: "One." Breathe out, and for the second name, say: "two," and so on until "ten," and then repeat. If you lose concentration at any point, kindly return your concentration to the breath.

2. BODY SCAN MEDITATION

The basic technique would be the body scan meditation, where you focus on the different body parts. It helps boost body consciousness and relax the muscles.

Practice: They must lie down or sit comfortably in a chair. For example, one can say something like, "Close your eyes and take a few deep breaths." First, pay attention to the toes and the feet and then gradually move up to the legs, stomach, chest, arms, and head. Notice any sensations or areas of tension. Breathe into those areas and release any tightness as you exhale. Spend a few minutes on each location.

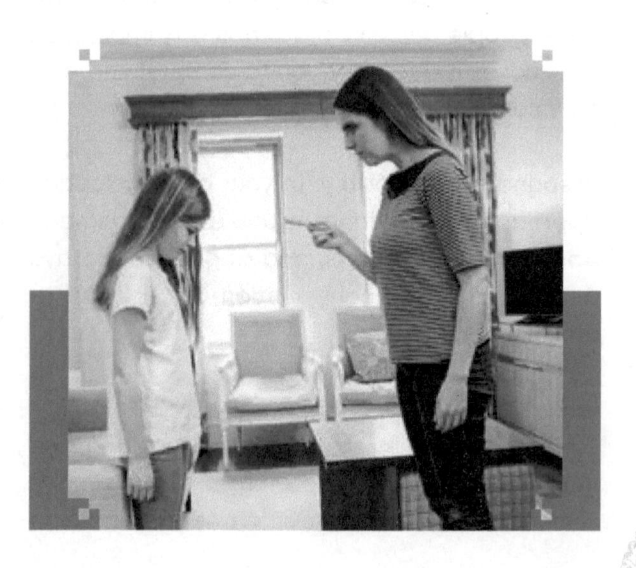

3. MINDFUL WALKING

Timed walking integrates the aspects of exercise with focused attention, which allows the person to regain attention to the present moment.

Practice: Locate an area where you can do this walking without the interruption of other people. As you walk, pay attention to the sensations of each step: the touch sensation that one gets from their feet when touching the ground, the music or beat that a dancer gets when dancing, or the setting in which the dance is being performed. Do not let your thoughts race; stay on the rhythm of walking and keep your attention on the sensations of this activity.

4. LOVING-KINDNESS MEDITATION

Loving-kindness meditation promotes positive affection towards the self and other people.

Practice: Get comfortable, relax in your sitting position, and close your eyes. Start with yourself and say such things in your mind: 'May I be happy, may I be healthy, may I be safe, may I have ease'. Progressively, expand these wishes to family and friends, people you meet daily, and enemies. Finally, free-flowing radiates loving-kindness to everyone unconditionally. Perform the practice for 10 to fifteen minutes each day.

5. GRATITUDE PRACTICE

Gratitude is one of the effective means of re-focusing on the constructive aspects of our lives, which leads to improved emotional health.

Practice: Take some time – even if it is a little- and write down things you are thankful for. You can try using a 'gratitude journal' where the last thing you have to do is write three to five things you are grateful for each day. In this step, you are required to concentrate on particular hours, days, months, or even years that are the most satisfying or give you a definite sense of happiness.

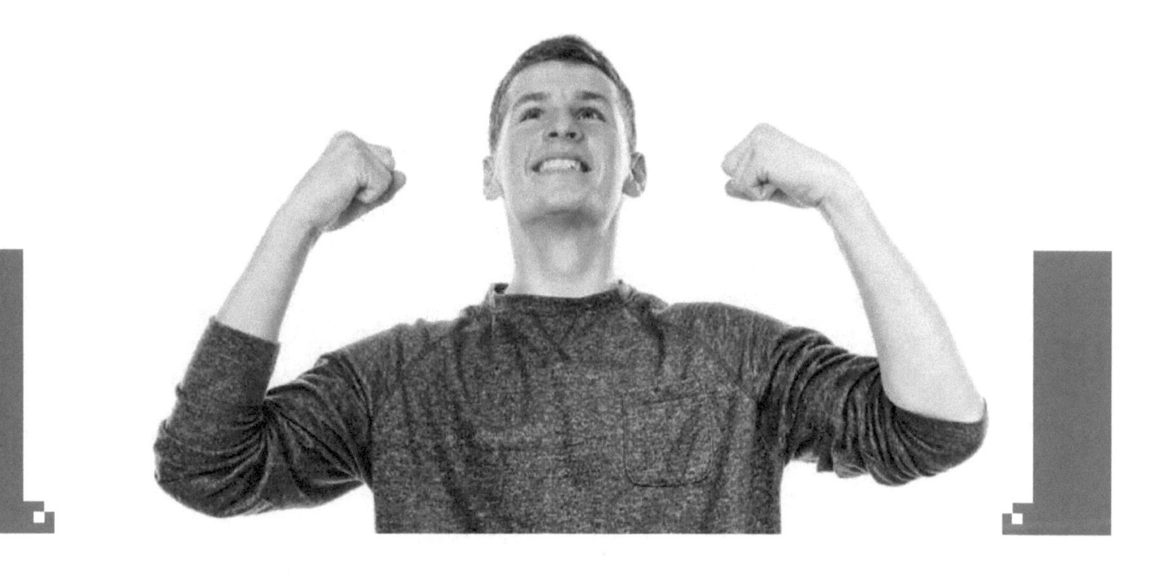

Chapter 6

Healing from the Past

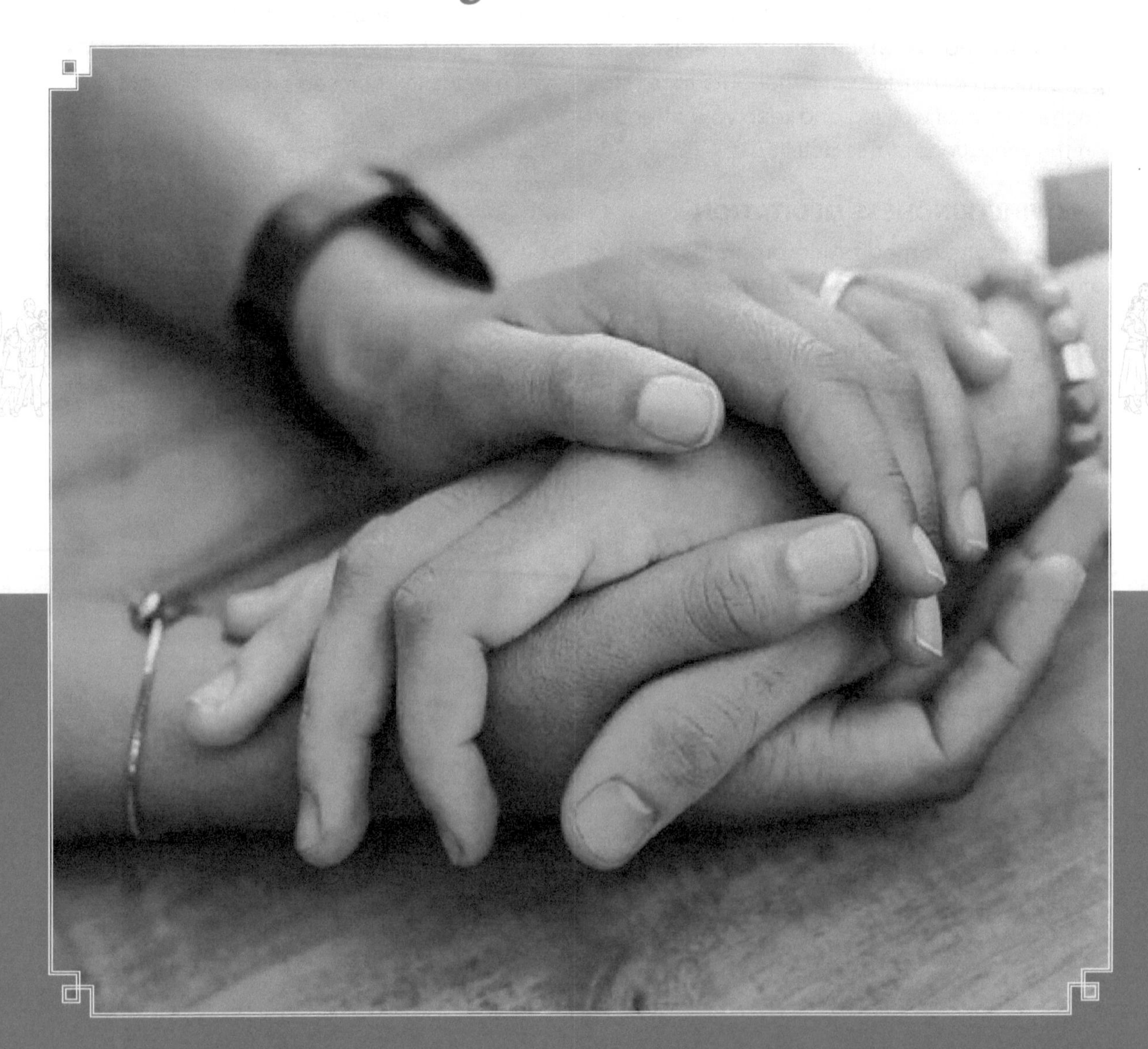

Getting over the trauma that comes with having toxic parents is a lifelong process, complete with tremendous change. It means acquiring the experience of placing oneself in a position where one has to face and live through fragments of painful memories that, having realized their influence on the present, one seeks to restore control and power over one's life. In their study, Harrison and Curtis argue that the psychological wounds which come from having distant, rejecting, and emotionally immature parents do not necessarily dissipate with time and can affect self-images, interpersonal relationships, and mental health in the caregivers' adulthood.

Looking at the various factors involved in healing from the past, this is the section to dissect the broad process delicately. It starts with the identification of the manifestations and consequences of toxic parents. This helps one to come out of the mental prisons created by such experiences, which form part of the emotional and psychological development of a person. We will investigate the typical toxic parenting style and traits as well as how such toxic patterns are reflected in children and how they affect them in adults, thereby increasing the levels of low self-esteem, lack of confidence, emotional disturbance and the like among them.

The Journey of Healing

Recovery from toxic parents is ongoing and complex because such parents are also continuous in their mistreatment. For many people, it is a gradual, ongoing and, to a certain extent, a lifelong concern that can take years to overcome. The rehabilitation process is about regaining one's right to honestly feel, setting up one's boundaries, and achieving inner harmony. In this chapter, you'll find descriptions of the several successive steps of the healing process and suggestions and practices helpful for this crucial phase of personal development.

Processing of anger and resentment at the workplace

Such feelings as anger and resentment are pretty frequent and, more than that, are pretty normal when one's parents are toxic. Such feelings are stressful and may lead to disastrous results if handled inadequately. Nevertheless, dealing with them is a mandatory step toward healing. Here are some tips as to how you can handle these or similar feelings:

To work through the overwhelmed anger and resentment, the initial stage involves bringing out the encouraged beliefs of the two emotions. Acknowledge that whichever way you look at it, it is normal for you to be angry. Such feelings should not be repressed or denied, but it is essential to recognize and experience them. Anger that is bottled up can also translate to raised levels of stress, depression and even some illness. Journaling can be influential if desired to counter and work through such emotions. Journaling has been found to help give angles on the causes of anger that an individual might not be aware of.

If, as a family member, you are facing the problem of anger, the first step is to find out where the anger is coming from. It is essential to know the root cause of anger so that appropriate action will be taken to prevent it. A self-assessment should then be done by recalling such incidences in the past or specific behaviors that have resulted in anger and resentment. This procedure can lead to recalling some unpleasant experiences, but this is essential for understanding better. The sources of anger may help you reduce its effect on your personal life and realize what your parents' actions have done to you.

Working Through Feelings of Anger and Resentment

There is a difference between 'constructive anger' and 'destructive anger.' It is expected to feel anger sometimes, but turning it on yourself or others negatively is not helpful. However, it is advised that you should look for productive ways to cope with such feelings of anger. Physical activity like exercising or playing sports can also assist in letting off steam, hence easing stress. Playing a musical instrument or drawing can also help to express the emotion, lessening the load of the feeling.

Learn to meditate and use other relaxation methods such as calming music, guided imagery, and so on. As will be discussed in this work, those mindfulness practices assist one in controlling one's mindset by making them calm, thus controlling emotions. Practical activities like meditation, breathing exercises and progressive muscle relaxation assist in calming down and decreasing the level of anger. Mindfulness can also assist in making a person more observant of their emotions and develop better ways of handling them.

COGNITIVE RESTRUCTURING

Cognitive restructuring requires you to dispute and alter the negative way of thinking that leads to anger and resentment. This is a CBT strategy that can assist one in adopting a less biased evaluation of the events in a particular situation. For instance, instead of saying 'My parents ruined my life", one can instead distil this to mean, "The terrible things that my parents inflicted upon me have had these effects on my life, but throughout it all, here I am surviving and thriving".

Emotional abuse is very damaging, and most of the offenders are the parents; it is essential to set and maintain boundaries to avoid more harm. Limitations are required to have a protective wall in your life and work to become a better person. This may involve limiting the interaction with your parents and expressing your needs and expectations, as well as being willing to back these up with consequences if your parents violate your rules. It is never wrong to set boundaries, as this is all about recognizing that one needs to care for and heal oneself

EMBRACE FORGIVENESS

Forgiveness is one of the most complex and must be wholly explained in the healing process. In this regard, asserting that forgiveness entails not condoning and excusing one's parents' toxic behavior is crucial. On the contrary, it involves the action of forgiveness to liberate oneself from anger and resentment derived from past incidents. Forgiveness, as people define it, is the process of removing oneself from such negativity and regaining one's state of mind. It can be a long process, and forgiving at your own pace when you are ready is certainly alright.

FOCUS ON PERSONAL GROWTH

Instead of channeling such negative concepts as anger or resentment into your life, please direct them to positive things such as personal development or improvement. Do things that make you happy and satisfied, and try to create an existence by your principles and plans

Remember that healing is a gradual process, and taking one step at a time is okay. You are not alone in this journey, and support is available to help you along the way.

Forgiveness: What It Is and What It Isn't

Healing entails several processes, of which forgiveness is a misunderstood and very important one. It is quite individual and can become the main factor that helps turn the page and heal from the harm caused by toxic parents. Here is what forgiveness is and is not, which would assist you in planning how to proceed in this sensitive phase of dealing with betrayal.

WHAT FORGIVENESS IS

1. Letting Go of Resentment: Apology requires letting go of the hold that the feelings of anger and resentment have on you. It is about washing oneself from the negative feelings that would chain an individual to past events. By letting go of such feelings, you will free yourself from allowing the positive feelings and experiences to come into your own.

2. Reclaiming Your Peace of Mind: So, forgiveness is the way to restore an individual's spirit and emotional state. Being angry and humble over things you could not change in the past is unproductive and unhealthy. It is possible to regain harmony in your life if you can forgive the people who wronged you.

1. Empowering Yourself: Through forgiveness, one regains power; thus, it can be viewed as empowering. It enables one to determine their emotional set instead of being a victim of their parents' actions. This shift element can make you feel more in charge and empowered in your life.

2. A Process: First, forgiveness is not an event but may take time, and second, different people may take different times to forgive. It entails accepting the fact that one is in pain, learning the effects of the pain, and releasing the related anger step by step. For such people, taking time before forgiving another for their mistakes is okay.

3. A Personal Choice: Forgiveness is a choice one makes for one's health. It is about the favorable decision to continue and begin the healing process. It is an option for one to choose joy and walk away from pain or stew in hatred day after day.

4. WHAT FORGIVENESS ISN'T

1. Condoning or Excusing Behavior: Do not lose the sense of forgiveness, thinking that it equals accepting or tolerating your parents acting like psychos. This is not a question of discounting or explaining the pain that they have inflicted. It becomes essential to admit the consequences of one's actions while at the same time learning to forgive.

2. Forgetting the Past: Forgiveness is not about forgetting the event but forgiving another person for wrongdoing against the one who forgives. It's about remembering in a way that doesn't bring more suffering to any of the subjects involved in the conflict. The concept here is to mend the brunt received by the psyche but not to wipe out memories of occurrences.

3. Reconciliation: However, forgiveness is not reconciliation by any chance. As to forgiveness, only some people need to reconcile with their parents, as seen from the various choices above. You can forgive someone without that person being in your life or having any contact with you. One should also ensure that one sets physical boundaries that should not be crossed so that one does not end up being abused again.

4. Immediate: It is worth underlining that forgiveness is not always spontaneous and happens right after. It's okay if it takes some time for you to get to a point where you begin to forgive the person. This is why rushing the process can be pretty detrimental. Take the time required to recover from a trauma.

5. Weakness: The act of forgiving is, therefore, not a sign of weakness as most people would want to believe. Forgiving others, particularly those who have caused a great deal of pain, requires strength and courage. That's essential to you and your healing: a strong and courageous woman who accepts herself as she is now.

Seeking Professional Help and Support

Recovery from toxic parent experiences can be a daunting task and perhaps draining. However, using strategies and support from friends and relatives is always helpful, and professional help will offer specific instructions depending on your circumstances and a stable plan for recovery. Counselling can be in different forms, such as in therapy form, counselling form, or even through support groups, which, in one way or another will assist you to gain back your health.

THE IMPORTANCE OF PROFESSIONAL HELP

Expertise and Guidance: Proper therapists and counsellors are qualified personnel with a deep focus on the mechanisms of maltreatment of a client emotionally and psychologically. They can give feasible recommendations that could be implemented in your case since they know the intricacies more than you do about your emotions and experiences. They can look past the symptoms, get to the root of the problem, and then solve it using the best practices. This is specific knowledge which can be indispensable if working with the multiple and often subconscious effects of toxic parenting.

A Safe Space: It is the type of treatment provided by professionals that allows a client to freely speak and share emotions without prejudice. Such a haven is vital in cases where one has emotionally charged issues to discuss, and it avoids situations when an individual is criticized for dressing a certain way or feeling a certain way. Here, you are protected and sensitive to face the ugly realities and uncomfortable facts and treat your suffering. The effectiveness of a therapist also lies in his ability to assure his patients and keep the information they share with them private. Understanding that someone will always be there for you without being judged will push you to explore the depths of your feelings.

Objective Perspective: The therapist helps explain the events in your life from a third person's view, giving you more insight. It can help you observe things that may have never caught your attention because you are involved. That is why I often notice that it is tough to be critical towards one's problematic aspects if one is intimately acquainted with them. A therapist can help you revitalize the situation and look at it from a different perspective that may not even cross your mind. This fresh perception can also help one discover what needs to be done and how to do it to progress in the healing process, thereby making better decisions for one's mental health care.

Structured Approach: Counselling or therapy is a focused way of getting better where the goal and how you will try to achieve it have been mapped out according to your problems. It may help to have a clear structure like this as it offers a form of framework and goals in healing. The patient and the therapist will agree on some objectives and plan how to reach them and what tasks must be accomplished to accomplish them. This plan can refer to any therapeutic processes and methods that may be individual to you. Having a clear map of what has to be done and when it has to be done may help and may, in one way or another, assist in making the healing process less daunting and more fruitful. It also enables one to check on the progress made with time, encouraging one to move on as one can see progress.

Therapeutic Techniques: CBT, EMDR, and More

Hiring a professional is the most significant action that needs to be taken when one has to face the difficulties of upbringing with toxic parents. Different counselling approaches can be essential in helping treat the emotional and psychological aspects, as seen in such incidences. Of these methods, CBT and EMDR are two of the most popular strategies categorized as evidence-based practices. However, several other working methods can be used to make it possible. Here is more information about such therapeutic techniques and ways they may help you recover.

COGNITIVE BEHAVIORAL THERAPY (CBT)

Understanding CBT:

A common type of therapy is cognitive behavioral therapy, which aims to change negative thinking patterns and actions. It is based on the premise that mental, emotional and behavioral responses are commonly linked; therefore, a change in the thinking process will automatically trigger changes in the feeling process and the behavioral response.

HOW CBT WORKS:

In CBT, a therapist assists a person in becoming aware of negative or irrational ideas and behaviors that cause discomfort. In different ways and employing different tasks, one is taught to confront and modify such thinking patterns with more appropriate, positive ones. CBT also uses behavioral components, like exposure therapy, whereby you are exposed to the stimuli that cause the condition and skills enhancement that helps you learn more appropriate ways of handling the problem.

BENEFITS OF CBT:

CBT has been proven helpful in the treatment of specific problems, such as cognitive-behavioral therapies, anxiety, major depression, and PTSD that many toxic parent victims may have. CBT, in particular, can be reported to give relief quite early because it does not attempt to explore the patient's personality but only examines current problems. It cultivates a course that equips you with ways and means to regulate your mind and thereby positively influence your psychological health.

Here is information on one therapy known as Eye Movement Desensitization and Reprocessing (EMDR).

Understanding EMDR: EMDR is a unique treatment method intended to focus on processing traumatic material in patients. It entails employing eye-muscle movement, among others, to assist the SH client in changing negative memories to more positive ones.

How EMDR Works: In EMDR, an individual is taken through a process where the therapist facilitates the recall of a traumatic event and, at the same time, engages the client in what is known as bilateral stimulation. It optimally reduces the emotional charge associated with the memory and, therefore, contributes to the reconsolidation process. The purpose is to decrease the aftereffects of trauma and enable you to put memory into a more adaptive form and less distressing one.

Benefits of EMDR: EMDR is most helpful in PTSD and other related disorders since it targets trauma as one of the leading causes of the disorder. This is because it can cause marked and fast changes in trauma symptoms in many clients and within several sessions less than that of conventional talk therapy. In contrast to other psychological therapies, EMDR provides a chance to directly recall and neutralize the severity of some past events, free of charge, and thus improve one's ability to cope with difficulties.

ADDITIONAL THERAPEUTIC TECHNIQUES

1. Psychodynamic Therapy: Psychodynamic therapy discusses behavior patterns and thinking outside a patient's conscious awareness. It seeks to reveal hidden intentions and grievances that remain in one's unconscious to enable them to be processed and healed. This approach is constructive in making one appreciate the effects of toxic parents and how they shape one's current interactions and outlook in life.

2. Dialectical Behavior Therapy (DBT): DBT is a CBT, which stands for dialectical behavioral therapy, accepting the best of change and changing the best of acceptance. Reported studies also show that the technique works best for persons with poor self-regulation emotions and clients with borderline personality disorder. DBT teaches skills in four key areas: Mindfulness, distress tolerance, emotion regulation and interpersonal effectiveness. They can assist in coping with extreme feelings, decreasing forms of self-harm, and enhancing relationships with other people.

3. Acceptance and Commitment Therapy (ACT): Acceptance and Commitment Therapy is a psychological intervention focusing on the need to accept distressing feelings and cognitions rather than attempting to eradicate or reduce them. Extending from it is acknowledging the importance of living a meaningful and values-based life when in emotional pain. ACT encompasses mindfulness exercises and focusing on specific behaviors that maximize psychological flexibility.

4. Mindfulness-Based Stress Reduction (MBSR): MBSR is an intervention developed to reduce stress using mindfulness meditation and yoga techniques. One of the things it instructs you to do is learn to be mindful of the present and not condemn yourself for what you think or feel. MBSR might be more helpful in addressing clients' anxiety, depression, and chronic stress due to toxic parenting.

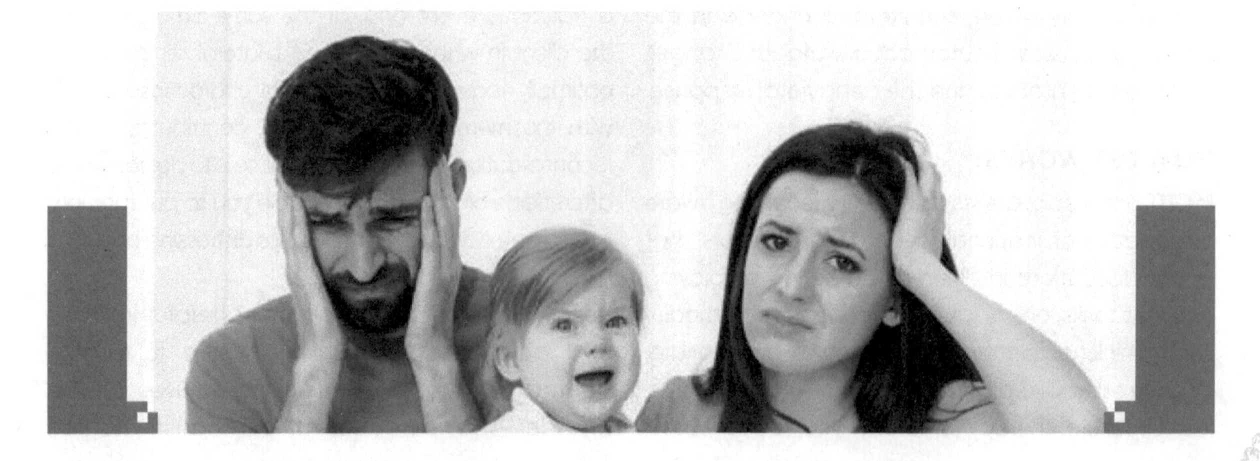

Chapter 7

Overcoming Guilt and Shame

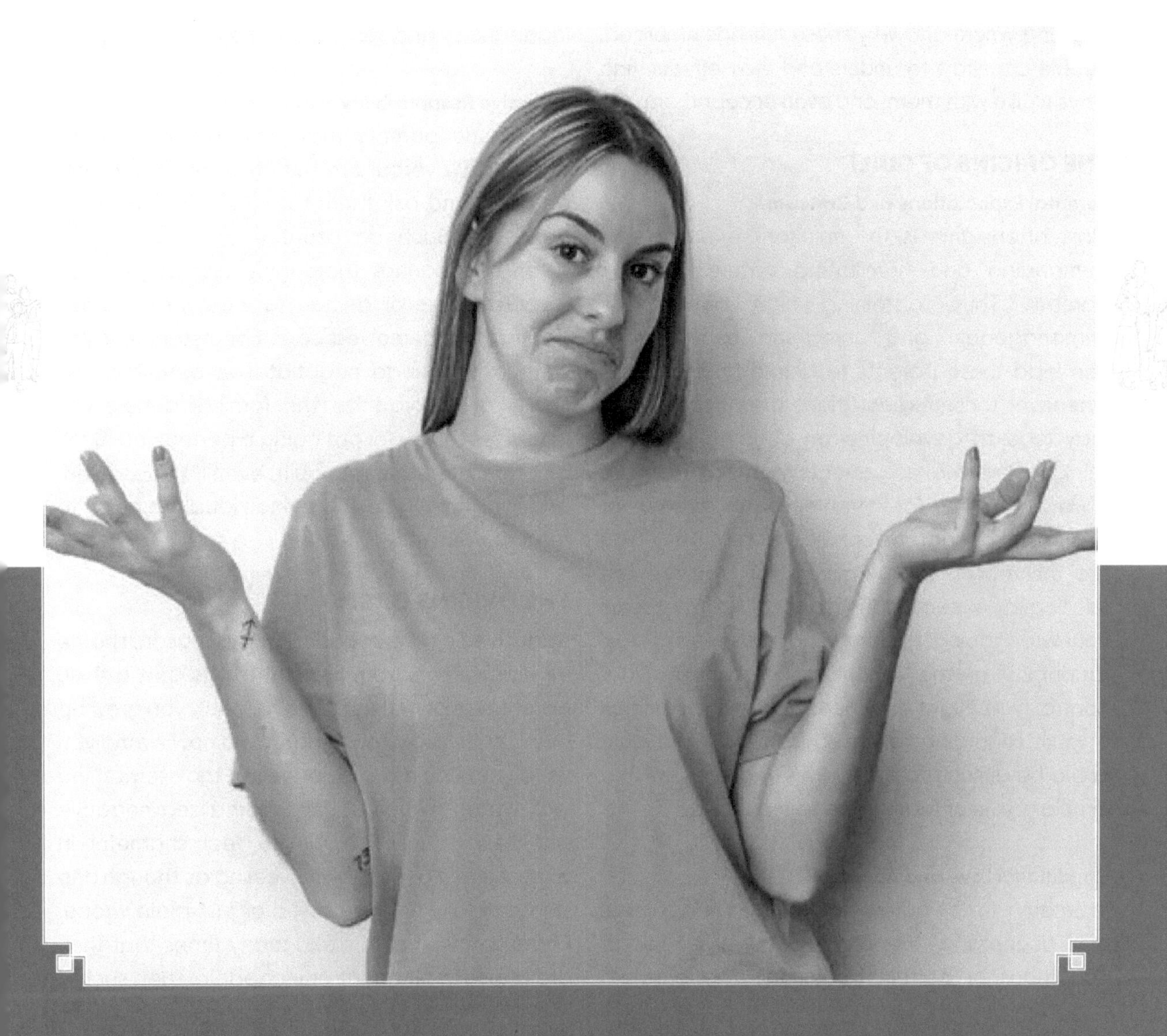

Understanding the Origins of Guilt and Shame

The feelings of guilt and shame are deep and differentiated, which emerge from the perspective of the developmental aspects of the personality of respondents with toxic parents. All these feelings will profoundly impact your sense of self, emotions, and interactions with others. It is, therefore, paramount to be able to know how guilt and shame begin to try and resolve the problem. Knowing where and why those feelings emerged, people can start to understand their effects, find ways to live with them, and even accept them.

THE ORIGINS OF GUILT

Parental Expectations and Criticism

Most often, guilt is the resultant effect of the demanding and humiliating nature of toxic parents. Thus, obtaining high but mostly unmanageable and unrealistic expectations can lead these parents to blame their children whenever those expectations are not met. This may lead to developing an ongoing mode of thinking that makes patients feel that they are always to blame for some feeling or action. For example, if a parent constantly tells you, 'You are the reason for my misery,' or 'You are not fulfilling my expectations,' to you, it translates as your wrongdoing. Regardless of these standards' rationality or the circumstances outside your control, you might experience profound feelings of guilt regarding failure. This internalized guilt could be difficult to deal with since it results in a circular cycle of blame and self-criticism.

Conditional Love and Approval

In many toxic parenting dances, happiness and acceptance depend on the given set of conditions or certain behaviors. The problem occurs when a child's value is seen based on what they do or accomplish or their obedience to their parents' expectations, thus qualifying the love they receive. The guilt resulting from the feeling that you are not worth much if you do not meet these conditions when you are reminded that this is who you are supposed to be can be overwhelming. This is because guilt results from the notion that one has failed to meet the perquisites that would bar them from deserving love or approval, leading to feelings of inadequacy and self-reproaches.

Excessive Responsibility

Narcissistic parents may emotionally or even practically overburden the child as if they were an adult and ask them to solve different family problems. Such an attitude can cause guilt when one cannot thoroughly discharge these responsibilities or decide to meet one's needs against the perceived care. For instance, if you were expected to negotiate on behalf of the family or to organize the family's duties, you would feel guilty for not doing a perfect job. Such a notion interferes with guilt, even if undeserved, and greatly hinders the individual's ability to tend to themself.

THE ORIGINS OF SHAME

Negative Self-Perception: For this reason, shame regularly stems from harmful things that a toxic parent tells or makes the child feel. If you grew up being criticized or constantly told how wrong you were, you could grow up feeling that something was wrong with you. This internalized negative self-view causes people to feel shameful in almost every aspect of life, feeling as though one is intrinsically untidy, flawed or just plain wrong. For example, if one is told many times that they are a disappointment or incapable, then such a message becomes carved into one's mind, and subconsciously, one starts accepting that there is something wrong with them as a person.

Rejection and Abandonment: In other aspects, rejection and abandonment by toxic parents help in the expression of shame. One may be rejected or made to feel unimportant repeatedly; hence, he tends to accept the invalidations as proof of his worthlessness. When one is often given the message that 'you are not good enough' or that 'no one can love you,' the outcome of such treatments is the formation of chronic shame. This internalized shame may present as self-conviction that one does not deserve to be loved, accepted or happy; a massive feeling of worthlessness would ensue.

Comparisons and Criticism: You may be constantly put down by toxic parents compared to other siblings or relatives, which often makes one feel ashamed. These comparisons and criticisms can fill one with a spirit of inferiority and give you the impression that you are a failure to society's expectations. For instance, the messages could be in the form of sibling or peer comparisons where one gets to conclude they are a failure or inadequate. These two are likely to lead to the deterioration of self-esteem and monitoring of others, with the back of shame affecting your self-worth and stress itself affecting you emotionally.

Knowing these roots aids in comprehending how such feelings unfolded and how they influenced an individual's life. Identifying guilt and shame with their origin to distinguish these feelings and start treating them is possible. This recognition is a good beginning in eradicating the ill consequences that may come with such emotions and the formation of a positive self-attitude.

Differentiating Between Healthy and Unhealthy Guilt

Guilt is a multifaceted emotion that can significantly guide moral behavior and foster personal growth. However, not all guilt is created equal. Differentiating between healthy and unhealthy guilt is crucial for understanding its impact on your well-being and making constructive changes.

HEALTHY GUILT

Motivates Positive Change:

Functional guilt is a guide to the conscience, assisting you in understanding if you have wronged other individuals or if your conduct is incompatible with your principles. It works as a driving force to change for the better and can push you into a desire to make up for your wrongdoings. For instance, if you offended someone and you regret your action, this type of guilt propels you to own up and try to amend for the wrong you have done; this, in the long run, builds better relations and growth of an individual.

Encourages accountability:

Compared to unhealthy guilt, healthy guilt is a normal or a positive thing since it indicates that a person owns up to their actions and is conscious of their impact on others. It speaks to your appreciation of the effect you have on other people as well as your accountability. This type of guilt results in constructive self-evaluation and searching for ways to ensure that one has not offended or done wrong. For example, shame for having failed to meet a particular obligation or realizing that you have not been as responsible as you should be can be a valuable signal to ensure you make changes for the better and be more accountable in the future.

PROMOTES EMPATHY:

Constructive guilt as it occurs along with the realization of the effects of one's actions on other people. Emphasizes ways of thinking that bring more civil sense into a person and make you or them have feelings for other people. Its practice benefits your associations by promoting understanding and appreciation of people's situations and feelings.

UNHEALTHY GUILT

Perpetuates Self-Blame:

Unhealthy guilt is different from it in that it refers to excessively blaming oneself and being overly critical of one when this is unnecessary due to the circumstances. It can be induced by such factors as setting unachievable goals or getting messages from parents that are toxic to the child. For instance, eating a piece of cake or gaining weight due to illness can make one constantly blame him or herself and make one feel unworthy. Such a practice will continue to make you blame yourself for the problems and overlook the root causes of the issues.

RESULTS IN PARALYZING FEAR:

Thus, unhealthy guilt can be expressed as a paralyzing fear of getting something wrong or of not being able to live up to expectations. This may translate into the belief that any time one fails or is subpar, it is shameful or that they are subpar in some way. For example, guilt for failure to achieve perfectionism in all areas of your life can make this fear stop you from taking risks or going for chances because you will always have the feeling of having failed in all the chances.

INTERFERES WITH SELF-CARE:

Unhealthy guilt often leads to neglecting your own needs and well-being in favor of meeting the demands or expectations of others. This guilt can be driven by a sense of obligation or a desire to avoid disappointing others, resulting in the sacrifice of your mental, emotional, or physical health. For example, feeling guilty about taking time for yourself and consequently overextending yourself to meet others' needs can lead to burnout and diminished self-care.

Strategies for Letting Go of Shame

Unpleasant feelings and self-conscious, apprehensive emotions have a profound influence on yourself and other individuals. It is usually traceable to one's background and self-biases and more so to those ovarian tyrants raised. Shame needs to be released for there to be changes and for one to create a healthier way of viewing oneself. Below are several detailed approaches to shedding shame and letting it go to improve one's quality of life and accept oneself.

1. AFFIRM YOUR FEELINGS

1. 1 Recognize the Source:

Therefore, the first thing that one needs to accept about shame is that it is a normal feeling that humans undergo due to childhood recollections and the poisonous ideologies from the environment one comes from. The positive effect of recognizing the source of shame is that it enables the distinction between those feelings and one's actual value and deals with them more effectively. For instance, if you experienced criticism or mockery from your parents or a close family member as a child, realizing that feelings such as shame originate from external factors instead of your failures or unworthiness can facilitate overcoming shame.

1. 2 VALIDATE YOUR EXPERIENCE:

There is a need to allow the self to feel and embody the shame without necessarily blaming the self for this feeling. This means acknowledging that you have feelings, and it is necessary to accept them when working on the case. To validate that a person's feeling stems from sexual assault, the therapist does not deny or diminish the experience but takes into account the feelings of shame inherent to the victim. This, in turn, is the first stage in fighting them because accepting oneself is the first key to overcoming such negative thoughts and emotions. Emotional validation means that you respect your feelings because they are honest and thus create the basis for recovery.

2. CHALLENGE NEGATIVE SELF-BELIEFS

2.1 Identify Core Beliefs:

Negative self-beliefs, such as inadequacy, worthlessness, or unworthiness, often feel shame. These core beliefs are usually formed based on past experiences or messages from toxic individuals. Identifying these negative beliefs is crucial for understanding how they contribute to your shame. For instance, if you believe you are inherently flawed because of past criticisms, recognizing this belief is the first step in challenging and changing it.

2.2 REFRAME NEGATIVE BELIEFS:

Recognizing the negative beliefs and replacing them with more optimistic and realistic ones is essential. Cognitive restructuring entails replacing negative messages that one usually arrives at with accurate messages that depict positive aspects in one's life, such as achievement, strengths, and value as a person. For example, during cognitive restructuring, if you think that you don't deserve love, challenge this thought by stating that everyone deserves love, including you. It's done to replace the feelings of shame with a healthier perception of oneself and the world.

3. PRACTICE SELF-COMPASSION

3. 1 Treat Yourself Kindly:

Self-compassion is a process of accepting oneself and practicing kindness about one's shortcomings, including the feeling of shame. Do not use bitter sentiments on yourself or, in other words, use kind words when talking to yourself. It is recommended that consumers talk to themselves like one would speak to a friend in distress. For instance, if you have made the wrong decision, instead of condemning yourself, try to encourage yourself and accept your mistake.

3. 2 ENGAGE IN SELF-CARE:

Make time for items that will enhance your overall health with an emphasis on self-esteem. Practicing personal interests, such as a hobby, exercise, or meditation, can benefit one's mental health. It explains elements of self-compassion rooted in self-care, whereby one consciously practices nurturing oneself. In other words, if an individual spends time in activities that offer them fun and relaxation, it will act as a form of self-entitlement that enhances their worth and virtue.

4. SEEK PROFESSIONAL HELP

4. 1 Therapy and Counseling:

One can seek professional help from a therapist or counsellor who deals with cases of shame and emotional trauma. Professional therapy is the encapsulation of a controlled environment where one can carefully look at why they feel shameful, find ways how to battle these shame triggers, as well as deal with other embedded problems. Counsellors are helpful as they can explain or give you an understanding of the issues behind shame and how to deal with them constructively.

5. PRACTICE VULNERABILITY

5.1 Share Your Story:

Letting people, you are close to knowing that you feel shameful will help you to deem shameful feelings less powerful. Telling your stories to friends or family members positively affects the feelings of shame and relieves the load on the sufferer. Safety enables one to open up and share their feelings, which helps them not feel so alone and start healing.

5. 2 Embrace Imperfections:

An essential part of managing shame is being able to accept and integrate people's imperfections. To manage expectations, you must understand that everyone has shortcomings and mistakes. Authenticity, through the acceptance of one's weaknesses and flaws, makes one feel more accessible and less ashamed. For instance, accepting that you are too human and that it is perfectly alright to mess up at times assists the individual in having a healthier perception of oneself.

Rebuilding a Positive Self-Image

Learning to accept ourselves is a process of recovery that helps a person change her perception of herself and heal herself. This process can be complicated if one has had their self-image defined negatively by toxic parentage or any other negative influences. Building and establishing a positive self-image is not just elevating one's self-esteem, but it is the act of daring and loving yourself after losing your worth and accepting the true worth that is in you.

These are the following approaches to assist you in the process of constructing a healthy self-image and experiencing optimism:

1. Self-schema determines a person's perception, including negative cognitions about the self. Hence, self-schema can be used as a tool to monitor and challenge negative perceptions about the self.

1.1 Recognize Negative Self-Talk: The process starts with identifying the impotent self-communication or the internal disability messages that affect the patient. These are usually rooted in earlier childhood or unfavorable environmental factors and may consist of negative attitudes toward the self or feelings of incapability. Several critical thoughts are bound to make you develop poor self-esteem, so give attention to those thoughts and how they influence your self-esteem. This is where one has to accept that these messages are a part of past hurt and are in no way a description of oneself.

1. 2 Reframe Negative Thoughts: These are some of the negative self-beliefs. Once you have recognized them, confront them, change their negative self-speaking, and substitute it with positive self-speaking. Challenge negative internal voices to reframe in the form of affirmative thoughts that embrace you and value you in positive ways. For example, instead of frequently having such negative thoughts as 'I am not worthy,' replace them with 'I have strengths and qualities that make me valuable.' This kind of change in the perception about one's self can help change one's perception dramatically for the better and help in gaining a positive body image.

1. 3 Set Realistic Expectations: One must also note that the goals should be coherent and realistic for the individual. Do not get sucked into the issue of perfectionism because it is destructive to one's self-esteem. Accept that everyone has some positives

and negatives, and it is impossible always to be perfect, and consistency will backfire. However, the targets you need to set in your case depend on your capabilities since you need to aim at what you stand to achieve midway. This approach creates a more lenient and positive attitude towards the self.

2. CULTIVATE SELF-COMPASSION

2. 1 Practice Kindness: It is the ability to be kind and understanding towards yourself as you would be to a good friend. In the same vein, if you get stuck with any issue or make a wrong decision, do not scold yourself but be encouraging. Admit that you are not perfect and that mistakes are a part of everyone's lives while keeping in mind that you need care and forgiveness. Acceptance of self-compassion may allow for healing the angry thoughts brought on by past criticisms and create a beneficial attitude toward oneself.

2. 2 Engage in Self-Care: Engage in behaviors that help fill your self-esteem and provide positive regard. Pursue well-being activities such as taking up a new hobby that will make you happy, exercising, taking a break, or going out with friends or family. Self-care is a sign of respecting the self and assists in reminding a person how valuable they are. Whenever you find time and engage in these recreational activities, you strengthen your self-perception and establish tranquility.

2. 3 Celebrate Achievements: Before we finish for the day or the week, ensure that you have taken time to acknowledge the goals that you have reached, however small they may be. It is important to celebrate them because it helps to maintain a positive self-identity and increases the level of confidence. Think about how far you've come and embrace your hard work because you have come a long way.

3. DEVELOP A GROWTH MINDSET

3.1 Embrace Learning: Adopt a growth mindset by viewing challenges and setbacks as learning and personal development opportunities. Understand that mistakes and failures are integral to growth and provide valuable lessons. Embracing this mindset helps you approach obstacles with resilience and optimism, seeing them as stepping stones rather than barriers to your self-worth.

3.2 Set Personal Goals: Establish personal goals that align with your values and aspirations. Setting and working towards goals gives you a sense of purpose and direction, contributing to a positive self-image. Break down larger goals into smaller, manageable steps and celebrate each milestone you achieve. This approach fosters a sense of accomplishment and reinforces your belief in your capabilities.

4. BUILD POSITIVE RELATIONSHIPS

4. 1 Surround Yourself with Supportive People: Focus on people with similar intercession and encourage you to progress. Being with such types of people provides successful self-images; thus, an individual's self-esteem is boosted. Focus on gaining like-minded friends and acquaintances, so you receive support and understanding that positively affects your emotional state.

4. 2 Seek Feedback: Ask for feedback from others who can give you an audited look at your skill set and personal flaws. Critique re-directs you to your strengths and skills, hence promoting self-erasure. Approach this feedback as a positive way of increasing self-confidence and strengthening self-image, while negative criticism can be a beneficial asset regarding individual progress.

4. 3 Set Healthy Boundaries: Set limits so as not to get into unhealthy interactions for your self-concept. Engaging in beneficial interactions concerning your welfare and avoiding toxic ones is advisable. By doing this, the client is in a position to accept that some things are beyond their control and, therefore, need to set limitations that will create a protective barrier around them, thus fostering a positive attitude about the self and positive emotions.

5. ENGAGE IN POSITIVE SELF-AFFIRMATION

5. 1 Practice Daily Affirmations: Designate a time in your calendar to affix positive things about yourself to your mind. An affirmation is a spoken or written word or phrase that has the foundation of one's character, personal values, and accomplishments in education and career. Being a program that is run daily, the constant use of such affirmations assists in overcoming negative thoughts and building confidence. Encourage the use of positive affirmations that are in harmony with one's wish list and personal principles when determining how one should perceive him or herself.

5. 2 Visualize Success: Pretend in your mind and visualize yourself attaining the objectives, then visualize yourself performing well in areas of your life. Visualization creates a picture of success in the sense of an individual; this is effective in increasing morale. When contemplating achieving goals and enjoying the positive consequences, a positive self-image is maintained, and hope is created.

5. 3 Focus on Strengths: It is essential to define and promote values such as strengths and talents. Valuing oneself builds up positive self-esteem when one accepts the qualities that distinguish oneself from others. What society sees in a negative light, one should see the qualities which make them feel valued and the good they do for society. This enables the building up of your confidence and the boosting of your self-esteem levels as you embrace your strengths.

6. ENGAGE IN SELF-DISCOVERY

6. 1 Explore Your Interests: Spend more time and energy on things that matter to you, and that you enjoy doing. Availing yourself to do other activities that keep you happy and satisfied assists in boosting the positive way of perceiving yourself and gives you purpose in life. Self-actualization enables one to access parts of one's self that give them worth, improving one's self-esteem.

6. 2 Reflect on Personal Values: Understand who you are and what you believe in. Knowing what is essential in one's life assists in achieving harmony between what one does and what one holds dear, thereby promoting feelings of relevance. If people act based on their values, then they maintain a positive self-conception, promote a high level of physical and psychological wellness, and essentially live out their authentic selves.

6. 3 Pursue Personal Growth: Promise yourself to continue growing, developing, and learning new lessons to be a better person. Do something that you consider meaningful as well as something that puts you out of your comfort zone. You feel more accomplished and, therefore, have positive feelings about yourself if you seek more business opportunities. Accept the process of station becoming the way to embrace the road to development and acceptance of one's potential.

7. PRACTICE MINDFULNESS AND SELF-AWARENESS

7. 1 Engage in Mindfulness Practices: It is recommended to practice mindfulness to learn to watch out for thoughts and feelings without any commentary. Meditation makes an individual's perception of self-more accepting or rational, thus buffering negative self-appraisals. Positive emotions are built through activities like meditation, deep breathing, and any activities that help one focus on the present and achieve a positive attitude towards the self.

7. 2 Increase Self-Awareness: Practicing mindfulness is one way of enhancing self-awareness, and one needs to check oneself regularly for thoughts, feelings, and actions. How people feel concurrently enables them to identify tendencies and factors that influence their self-image. The element of personal growth consists of self-reflection; it also aids in the negation of negative attitudes towards oneself, promoting a healthy dose of self-appreciation.

7. 3 Use Journaling: You should maintain your journal to record and analyses your thoughts and emotions. Writing in the journal enables one to have a record of one's progress and develop an understanding concerning self-esteem. Journaling your experiences and personal growth promotes awareness and remembrance of the changes that need to be made, hence the process of building a new self-image.

In this respect, modifying self-image to be positive entails recognizing negative self-beliefs. This enables you to accept yourself and start a new life of having worth through self-acceptance, hence attaining personal strength.

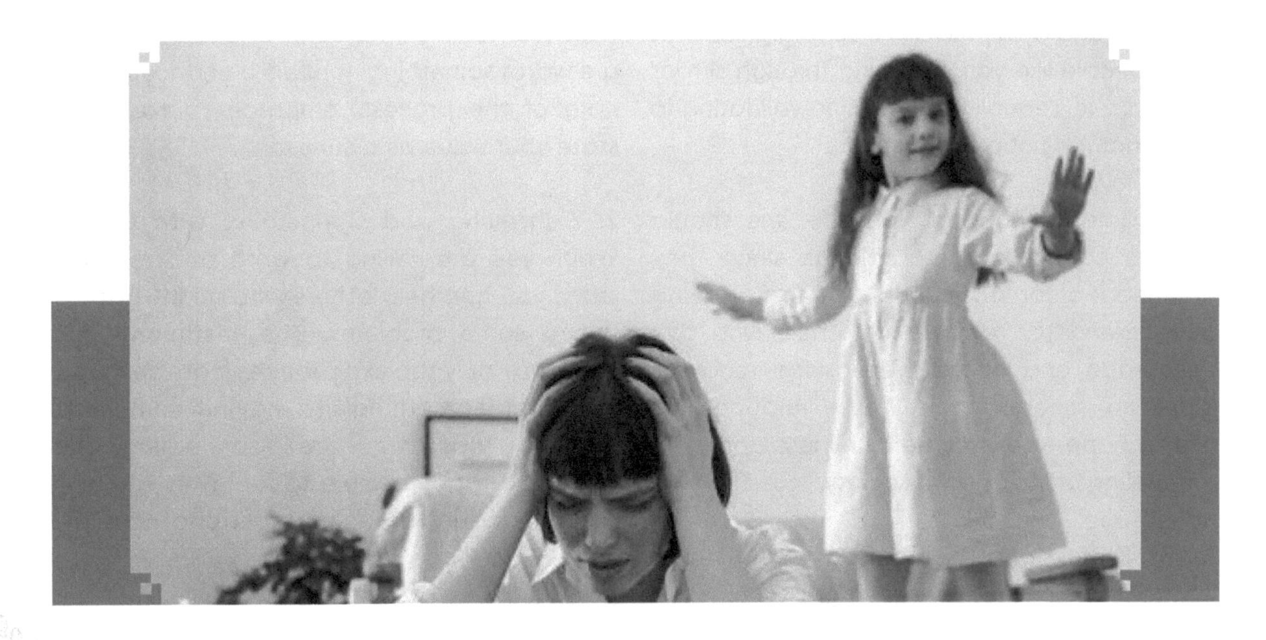

Seeking Support and Sharing Your Story

Becoming and getting support alongside telling one's story are crucial steps on the way to healing and reconstructing a healthy self-image, especially if a person was the subject of toxic child-rearing or suffered other forms of abuse. It mainly involves the social process of interacting with other members and being able to give an account of one's experiences, which offers excellent emotional comfort, acceptance, and understanding. This is why asking for help and narrating one's story is crucial, as well as some tips on how to ask for help and tell your story.

1. HOW SAYING YOU NEED HELP IS SUPER STRONG

1. 1 Emotional Relief and Validation: Seeking help gives a platform to vent out and acquire encouragement and understanding from others. Talking about issues one is facing with similar or like-minded people may help ease a burden and make one feel that somebody cares. Just like 'Here and Now', the aim is to recognize that other people like you are going through similar problems; it is equally calming and validating to know that it is not a fight alone.

1. 2 Building a Support Network: One should have a caring family or friends since they are needed for occasional comfort. Having good friends or relatives or others who can encourage and accept you during recovery plays an important role. These relationships offer a hope to overcome loneliness and gain the feeling of inclusion in society.

1. 3 Professional Guidance: Counseling with the help of a practicing psychiatrist, psychologist or counsellor is relevant because it is individualized. Trained people need to share advice, ways of dealing with the problem, and treatment methods with you. The problem is that with their help, one can work on oneself and eliminate profound problems rooted in one's subconsciousness.

1. 4 Creating Accountability: Such forums as the support group or a therapy session are most useful in enabling you to arrive at the goals you need to achieve in the recovery process. Telling others about your experiences makes it easier for you to remain focused on your development because the information you have shared is already out there. Indeed, this external support can help reinstate your morale and determination to go on.

2. SHARING YOUR STORY

2. 1 Finding Your Voice: When you tell your story, you discover your true identity and control over the kind of narrative created for you. Putting them into words can be transformative, a way of taking back control and saying you are worth something. It offers a chance to take note of the process, embrace yourself, and state your value as a survivor.

2. 3 Inspiring and Connecting with Others: When you are willing to write and tell your story, you can help others who might also be facing some problems. The testimony and the truth of your experiences can be hope, approval, something like having someone's back for those who are also healing. This link encourages people to feel they are with like-minded individuals and strengthens the concept of hope for recovery.

2. 4 Encouraging Open Dialogue: The storytelling fosters discussions that otherwise would not be possible and an interaction that helps to demystify the mystique generally associated with the state of mental health or even the general well-being of an individual. Getting into a dialogue and sharing the story can help create a more tolerant culture and improve the world. This openness can also allow other people to come out and share their experiences in society, hence increasing the rate of compassion.

3. STRATEGIES THAT HELP IN SEEKING SUPPORT

3. 1 Reach Out to Trusted Individuals: Search the people you know, including your friends, close relatives and role models, to talk to and share with them, incredibly when depressed. Be categorical and, most importantly, honest when communicating your emotions or recounting your story. Being around friendly people helps one open up and discuss the issues that they are going through.

3. 2 Join Support Groups: One may participate in the groups or communities that pertain to their circumstances. Beneath the structure of support groups, it offers a friendly environment where you can relate to people facing similar challenges. Such groups provide a place for people to share stories, get ideas, and be encouraged.

3. 3 Seek Professional Help: Speak to mental health workers who specialize in the areas of abuse and other incidents that have happened to you. A professional therapist or counsellor can provide individualized advice and psychotherapy methods on how you shall be able to overcome this process. It offers professional assistance, which can be very helpful because it will come from an independent source different from the ones you are dealing with daily. You can open up to this person, and they will be able to advise you based on their expertise.

3. 4 Engage in Peer Support: Join support groups or be active in the mentorship forums where you can also help out. Being in the company of people in similar circumstances enables one to explain to others and, in return, be comforted by the same people, besides gaining from what other people have to tell and offer in similar situations.

This process includes behavior changes and effective understanding to empower personnel and enhance personal resourcefulness to cope with stressors.

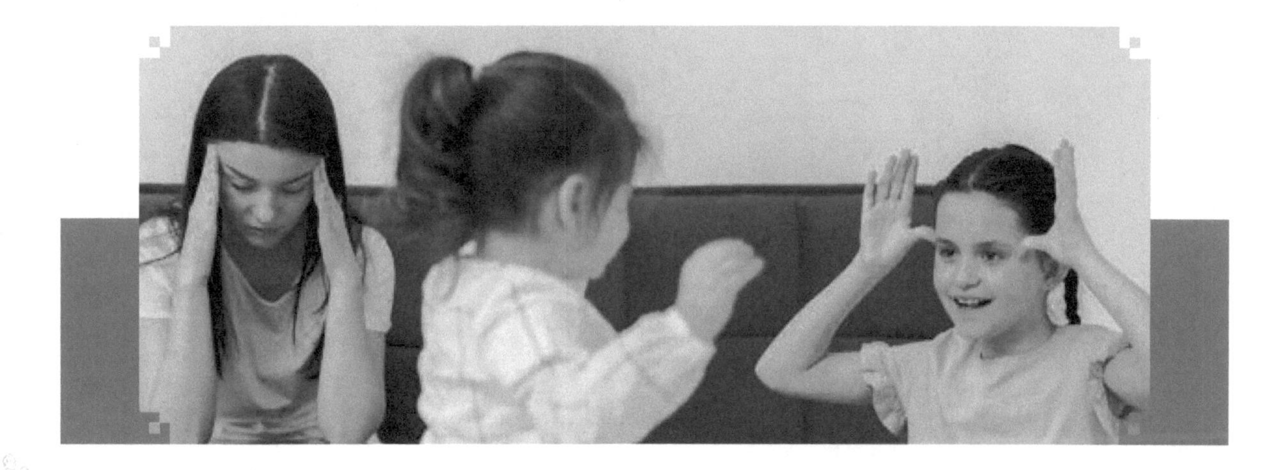

Chapter 8

Building Resilience and Inner Strength

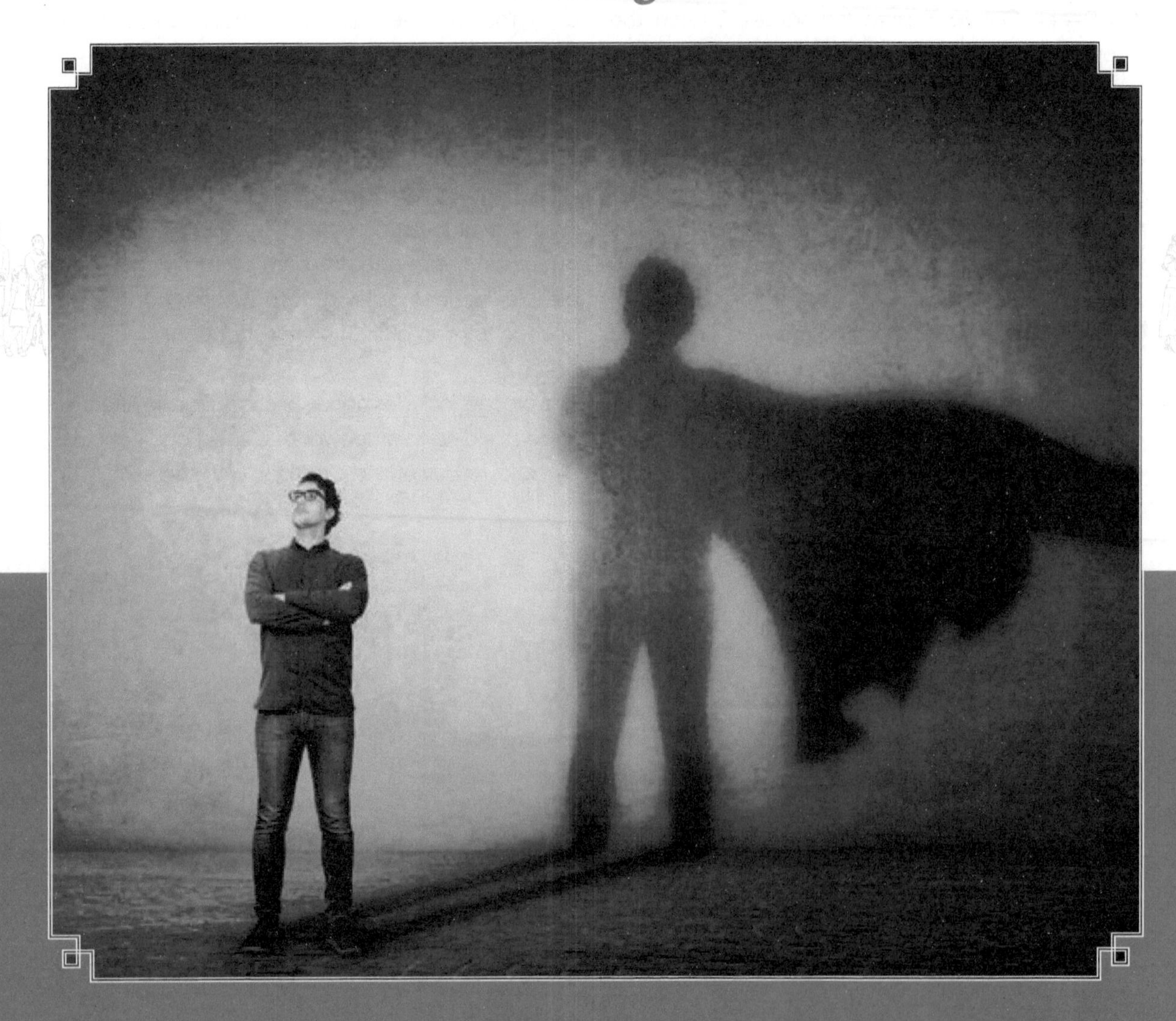

The development of personal resources is a milestone in one's character and self-therapy that is critical to achieve if faced with toxic parents or other types of emotional trauma. Coping and recovery after stress are the measures or one's ability to effectively cope with challenges and remain determined to overcome them in spite of various circumstances. On the other hand, inner strength deals with qualities that discriminate to get what is required in times of adversity, for instances, courage, determination and self-belief to face adversities. Acquiring these qualities is not a mere process of suffering; it is the process of suffering constructively and emerging with new discoveries.

Developing a Resilient Mindset

To sum it up, implementing personal strategies contributes to constructing a coping framework and nurturing a solid core. It is essential to understand that resilience is not the permanent characteristic of the human being but rather the result of the ongoing process of practices in action. It includes coping with problems, returning from a disaster, and sustaining optimism and a mission. Resilience enables one to conduct themselves in a manner that allows one to proceed with simple pleasures despite adversities. Here's a deeper look at how you can develop and nurture a resilient mindset: Here's a deeper look at how you can develop and nurture a resilient mindset:

1. CULTIVATE A GROWTH MINDSET

1. 1 Embrace Challenges as Opportunities: By getting a growth factor culture, the tendency is to see a setback or a difficulty as something that can be overcome rather than something that can only be endured. Instead of concentrating on the situation's challenges, focus on creating an opportunity for experience and skills acquisition. This view allows you to solve challenges without being overwhelmed by the problem or giving up easily.

1. 2 Learn from Failure: Always remember that perfection is not achievable, and getting things wrong sometimes is okay in learning. When you encounter problems, see what went wrong and what changes you could make. Learn to accept failing as a normal process of getting to success and capitalize on the experiences by growing coping mechanisms.

1. 3 Focus on Effort and Progress: Stop focusing on the results you want to achieve and increase your effort and work. Celebrate that you have worked, struggled, and done your best to face the journey in life, even if the result is not what you expected. This focus on effort helps build resilience since effort is more within the individual's control and thus increases the likelihood that the individual will persist through difficulties.

2. DEVELOP EMOTIONAL REGULATION SKILLS

2. 1 Practice Mindfulness: Awareness is the ability to be conscious of the present moment, of one's thoughts and emotions and experiencing them without passing any judgment. Meditation and deep breathing, among other things related to mindfulness, assist any person in handling stress and ensuring emotional stability. Meditation, in particular, is taught to be done at least fifteen minutes each day or at least twice a day because it trains one's mind to maintain focus during pressure situations.

2. 2 Use Cognitive Restructuring: One of the significant components of cognition stress reduction is cognitive restructuring, in which the negative patterns of thinking that cause stress and anxiety are flagged and combatted. Learn to challenge and replace negative thoughts with more realistic and helpful ones. It assists you in staying more optimistic in your perception and thus approaching events in life with more strength.

2. 3 Build Emotional Awareness: Get acquainted with the emotions you get and the conditions that cause stress. Recognizing emotional patterns serves as a means of regulating one's reactions to them and not getting carried away. Emotional awareness is a critical component of resilience, enabling you to navigate challenges with a more precise and more composed mindset.

3. STRENGTHEN PROBLEM-SOLVING SKILLS

3. 1 Break Down Problems: When a student encounters a problem, they should try to decompose it into several subtasks. Such an approach reduces the overall complexity of the problem and permits one to devise a plan of attack on the parts in an orderly manner. This way, problems are solved in a progressive manner, which enhances one's confidence in handling problems and improves problem-solving resilience in as much as it is comprehensive in approach.

3. 2 Develop Action Plans: Develop the strategies for the objectives and problems in your undertaking. Include the actions that are required and the time needed to accomplish them. By having a plan, you are well-directed and thus feel like you are in charge and can easily overcome challenges that come your way.

3. 3 Seek Solutions, Not Just Problems: Concentrate more on the solutions than worrying about the problems. Switch your thinking orientation from the negative aspect of a situation to the positive aspect of what can be done to transform or fix it. This then poses the problem of how to prevent these things from happening so as to encourage you to tackle issues proactively and combat them before they affect you.

4. FOSTER SOCIAL SUPPORT

4. 1 Build a Support Network: Maintain friends and family who have a good understanding and can appreciate your efforts and provide advice and help for your needs. Social support is emotional support and helps resolve problems, increasing one's coping capacity and personal strength.

4. 2 Seek Feedback and Guidance: Use time for constructive criticism from mentors, advisors, or close friends. They can provide you with the right perspective, assist you in making the right decisions, and consolidate your strength and ability to solve problems.

4. 3 Share Your Experiences: Especially when people can discuss their difficulties and problems – this can help both from the point of view of the internal state and the interactions between people. One aspires to seek others' support, advice, and care, promoting resilience by expressing thoughts and developing feelings.

5. MAINTAIN A POSITIVE OUTLOOK

5. 1 Practice Gratitude: Make gratitude a part of your everyday activities by making it a point to look at the brighter side of life. This thinking aims to bring you from the things that are missing towards the things that are present and available; in essence, it encourages a positive change of attitude.

5. 2 Visualize Success: Daydream in a positive manner, that is, visualize yourself to be able to overcome barriers and succeed. It is empowering and motivating to imagine positivity and positive results, strengthening the person's resolution.

5. 3 Celebrate Small Wins: It is also appropriate to take time and recognize the accomplishment of tasks, no matter how minor the accomplishment

may be. Encouraging yourself applauds you for your achievements, creating confidence to deal with the next obstacle encountered. Happiness promotions further develop a positive self-identity and strengthen one's optimal levels of coping.

Coping Strategies for Difficult Times

When life gets tough, it is stressful and can cause emotional wear and tear if one is struggling to cope with the impact of toxic people or any other hardship they have faced. Stress can be diminished, and proper coping strategies can enhance one's emotional stability and resilience. These should be strategies that can help you see through bad times and come out of them more robustly. Here's a comprehensive guide to various coping strategies that can help you navigate challenging times: Here's a comprehensive guide to various coping strategies that can help you navigate challenging times:

1. DEVELOP HEALTHY ROUTINES

1.1 Establish a Daily Routine: Establishing an organized schedule gives the one planning the schedule the much-needed discipline, which can prove very helpful during unsettled moments. Ensure that you incorporate some activities that touch on the health of the body, the emotions, and the mind, i.e., meals, exercise, and rest time, respectively.

1. 2 Incorporate Self-Care Practices: Self-care should also be a priority, meaning that one should do things that help to rejuvenate the body and the mind. These include interests, books, bathing, or just being outdoors, which should be considered enjoyable among the three subjects. Caring for oneself decreases stress, thus improving the quality of an individual's life.

1. 3 Maintain a Balanced Diet and Exercise Routine: Incorporation of adequate and appropriate nutrition in the diet and regular exercise can cause moods and energy levels to improve. Exercise has many benefits, including releasing feel-good hormones called endorphins to help the body handle stress.

2. PRACTICE MINDFULNESS AND RELAXATION

2.1 Engage in Mindfulness Meditation: Mindfulness meditation is one of the types of meditation that allows individuals to pay attention to what is happening at the moment without having to make any evaluations. Meditation also has implications in relieving anxiety in that it assists in developing ways of relaxing as well as gaining insight. Mindfulness can be promoted using techniques that include deep breathing, guided imagery, and a body scan.

2. 2 Try Progressive Muscle Relaxation: PMR is a technique where one tightens and then releases the muscles gradually to eliminate physical tension and stress. It enables customers to recognize physical rigidity and leads to general relaxation.

2.3 Explore Yoga and Stretching: Yoga combines physical postures, breathing exercises, and meditation to promote relaxation and reduce stress. Gentle stretching exercises can also help alleviate bodily tension and improve your sense of well-being.

3. CONNECT WITH SUPPORT NETWORKS

3. 1 Reach Out to Friends and Family: Similarly, discussing the situation with friends and relatives may help get some support or receive necessary materials. Telling your story to friends and family will help you not feel so alone and that people understand what you are going through.

3. 2 Seek Professional Support: It is always helpful to seek the advice of mental health workers, including therapists or counsellors, when in a dilemma. One can get support on dealing with such feelings from professionals, which will enable an individual to handle such feelings properly.

3. 3 Join Support Groups: Being involved in support groups or forums dedicated to your difficulties can help you feel you are not alone. These groups allow people with similar challenges to discuss their experiences, learn from one another, and be encouraged.

4. APPLIES COGNITIVE AND BEHAVIORAL INTERVENTIONS

4. 1 Challenge Negative Thought Patterns: A stressor is a condition that triggers the stress response; cognitive stressors involve negative thoughts that elicit stress; cognitive stressors include identifying and combating negative thinking that leads to stress and anxiety. Cognitive restructuring is another helpful technique that allows you to put in the right mindset and dismantle negative thinking. Cognitive restructuring works to change the way one thinks and is significant in building up the individual's emotional strength.

4. 2 Set Realistic Goals and Break Tasks Down: Having reasonable objectives and approaches and dividing elaborated tasks into estimable activities may also assist in decreasing the level of anxiety. Emphasize achieving one step at a time; do your best at that particular step and be happy when at that step.

4. 3 Practice Problem-Solving Skills: Set up and integrate particular techniques to solve specific issues you are struggling with. Assess the given situation, brainstorm the possible ways to respond, and make a plan of action. Problem skills give one a feeling of control and the ability to manage challenges.

5. ENGAGE IN POSITIVE ACTIVITIES

5. 1 Pursue Hobbies and Interests: Spend time doing things that interest you and are helpful to your soul. Engaging in hobbies and interests helps one focus on stress and generally makes one a better person. Whether it's painting, gardening, playing a musical instrument, whatever it is, find what makes you happy.

5. 2 Practice Gratitude: One could introduce gratitude into their daily schedule by focusing on the positive things that they have in their life. One can write down things for which one is grateful or take a few minutes each day to think about what one is thankful for to focus one's mind on things that can bring positivity.

5. 3 Volunteer or Help Others: Helping others [or volunteering] can help someone feel helpful and needed. Anonymously participating in your community or helping those in need can make you feel less lonely and happier. Thus, it is good to volunteer at such institutions.

The Role of Self-Compassion in Building Strength

Self-compassion is, therefore, vital in constructing one's resilience, including when the person has gone through lots of emotional needs or has been through lots of emotional suffering. Self-care is the process of taking care of oneself in a way that is similar to how one would care for a good friend. Self-compassion can help handle stress and life lessons, enhance resilience, and transform one's attitude towards the self. Here's how self-compassion contributes to building strength and resilience:

1. UNDERSTANDING SELF-COMPASSION

1.1 What is Self-Compassion? It is the ability to show compassion and understanding towards oneself in conditions such as failure, personal hardship, or suffering. It includes acknowledging the client's self-inflicted pain and embracing it without trying to fix or pass judgment. Self-compassion consists of three core components: self-compassion, other compassion, and present hedonism.

1. 2 Self-Kindness: Self-compass entails being kind to yourself instead of hounding yourself with criticism like you would with other people you do not like. Self-compassion applies when one may experience difficulties or fail; here, you are supposed to be kind to yourself rather than dwell on mistakes.

1. 3 Common Humanity: This reality indicates that everyone, no matter how much they strive to be perfect, is bound to go through one or more trying moments. If other people experience fish and amphibians as annoying as you and occasionally make mistakes, everyone can feel alone and guilty.

1. 4 Mindfulness: Mindfulness intentionally pays attention to feelings and events. It helps you to describe your emotions and develop an attitude regarding them, which does not include judgment because you learn how to relate to thoughts and feelings.

2. BENEFITS OF SELF-COMPASSION

2. 1 Enhances Emotional Resilience: Appreciation is vital in boosting one's emotional security since self-compassionate people have kind words to say to themselves during tough times. While self-criticism involves excluding hope and negative self-evaluation, self-compassion involves taking a calm and accepting attitude towards challenges, which, in turn, helps in overcoming them.

2. 2 Reduces Stress and Anxiety: It has been found that people who are compassionate towards themselves are likely to be stressed and anoxic as compared to those who are not. Self-compassion puts down the overwhelming self-criticism, allowing others to have more positive emotions and making them stronger.

2. 3 Promotes a Positive Self-Image: Self-compassion assists in developing positive self-esteem since it entails behavioral techniques of questioning negative self-images and practicing self-kindness. If one understands oneself gently and positively, the image of oneself in the mind is much healthier.

2. 4 Encourages Personal Growth: A healthy space for change and cultivating one's character is fostered by agreeing to self-compassion. It allows you to persevere and keep going because instead of getting upset with yourself for what you could not do, you understand why it was impossible and how to avoid getting to the same point again.

3. PRACTICING SELF-COMPASSION

3. 1 Develop a Self-Compassionate Mindset: First, it is necessary to identify negative thoughts and realize that they are irrational and unfair to oneself. Correct negative self-estimation with a less critical view of oneself. Remember, while facing particular ordeals, it is okay not to be perfect and that you need and deserve support and understanding.

3. 2 Use Compassionate Self-Talk: They should practice using sure and kind words when speaking to themselves. Use positive and encouraging self-talk instead of using negative self-talk and calling one's name. For instance, replace the following negative thinking and self-talk: "I am such a failure" with "I did my best, and it's okay to make mistakes.

3. 3 Engage in Self-Compassionate Actions: Engage in purposeful behaviors that promote your care and support your healthy development. This can range from scheduling free time, doing things that make you happy, and caring for your body and mind.

3. 4 Practice Mindfulness and Meditation: CBT should be integrated with MBIs like mindful breathing and other exercise forms to increase the patient's level of self-reflection and self-compassion. Mindfulness assists in thinking about the thought processes in a more accepting way, while self-compassion meditations encourage the process of being gentle towards oneself.

3.5 Embrace Your Humanity: Acknowledge that being human involves experiencing joys and struggles. Accepting your imperfections and recognizing that everyone faces challenges helps foster a sense of shared humanity and reduces feelings of isolation.

4. INTEGRATING SELF-COMPASSION INTO DAILY LIFE

4.1 Create Self-Compassion Rituals: Establish rituals or practices that reinforce self-compassion daily. This could include starting or ending your day with affirmations, keeping a gratitude journal, or engaging in regular self-care activities.

4.2 Surround Yourself with Supportive Influences: Build relationships with people who uplift and encourage you. Surrounding yourself with supportive individuals reinforces your self-compassionate mindset and provides a network of positive reinforcement.

4.3 Set Realistic Expectations: Set achievable goals and expectations for yourself, recognizing perfection is not attainable. Embrace progress and effort rather than focusing solely on outcomes.

4.4 Seek Professional Guidance if Needed: If you find it challenging to practice self-compassion or address underlying issues, consider seeking support from a mental health professional. Therapy can provide additional tools and strategies for cultivating self-compassion and addressing self-criticism.

In summary, self-compassion is a powerful tool for building strength and resilience. Treating yourself with kindness, understanding, and acceptance fosters emotional resilience, reduces stress, and cultivates a positive self-image. Practicing self-compassion helps you navigate challenges more efficiently and promotes personal growth and well-being. Embracing self-compassion as a core aspect of your healing journey will enhance your ability to cope with difficulties and enrich your overall quality of life.

Finding Meaning and Purpose After Trauma

Experiencing trauma can shake the very foundation of your sense of self and purpose. It often leaves you grappling with a profound sense of loss and confusion. However, finding meaning and purpose after trauma is not only possible but can lead to significant personal growth and renewed vitality. This journey involves exploring and redefining what matters most and discovering a path that aligns with your values and aspirations.

First, it is crucial to acknowledge the trauma and its impact on your life. Recognizing and validating your feelings of pain and loss are essential steps in moving forward. Accepting the reality of your experiences helps you address them more effectively and opens the door to healing.

Reflecting on your core values and beliefs is a powerful way to begin finding meaning. Trauma often shifts your perspective on life, making it an ideal time to reassess what truly matters to you. Understanding your values can align your actions and goals with what resonates deeply, providing direction and motivation.

Setting meaningful goals that reflect your values can foster a sense of purpose and fulfilment. Focus on goals that enhance your well-being and contribute to a greater understanding of purpose. These goals provide direction and help you channel your energy into satisfying activities.

Engaging in self-discovery is another crucial aspect of finding meaning. Explore your strengths, passions, and interests to understand yourself better. This deeper self-awareness can reveal new paths and opportunities that align with your sense of meaning.

Connecting with others is also crucial in this journey. Building and nurturing relationships can provide a sense of belonging and support. Share your experiences with trusted friends or family members, and seek out communities or support groups where you can connect with others who have faced similar challenges.

Helping others can create a profound sense of purpose and fulfilment. Volunteering or supporting those in need allows you to find meaning through acts of kindness and service, fostering a sense of connection and value.

Professional guidance can be invaluable as you navigate this process. Working with a therapist or counsellor can offer insights and tools for exploring and understanding your experiences more deeply, helping you find meaning and purpose after trauma.

Embracing personal growth is a natural outcome of this journey. Trauma can lead to significant changes in your perspective and strengths. By approaching these changes openly, you can develop new skills and strengths that contribute to your sense of purpose.

Practicing self-compassion is essential throughout this process. Treat yourself with kindness and understanding as you navigate the challenges of finding meaning. Self-compassion helps you accept your struggles and celebrate your progress, fostering a positive and resilient outlook.

Finding joy and fulfilment in life's activities is also essential. Engage in hobbies and passions that bring you happiness. Rediscovering what makes you feel alive and content can enhance your overall well-being and sense of purpose.

Creating a vision for your future that incorporates your newfound sense of meaning and purpose can guide your decisions and actions. This vision helps you focus on what matters most and supports your ongoing journey toward healing and fulfilment.

In summary, finding meaning and purpose after trauma involves acknowledging your experiences, reflecting on your values, and setting goals that align with your aspirations. By connecting with others, helping those in need, and embracing personal growth, you can discover renewed vitality and a more profound sense of purpose. Integrating meaning into your life fosters resilience and supports your journey toward healing and well-being.

Techniques for Sustaining Long-Term Resilience

Building resilience is an ongoing process that requires conscious effort and dedication. While the journey towards resilience begins with recognizing and addressing challenges, sustaining it involves implementing strategies that reinforce your ability to cope with and thrive despite adversity. Here are critical techniques for maintaining long-term resilience:

1. Cultivate a Growth Mindset: Adopting a growth mindset—believing that your abilities and intelligence can be developed through effort and learning—is essential for long-term resilience. This mindset helps you view challenges as opportunities for growth rather than insurmountable obstacles. Embrace setbacks as chances to learn and improve, and approach problems with curiosity and perseverance.

2. Develop Strong Support Networks: Building and nurturing supportive relationships is vital for strength and encouragement. Surround yourself with people who uplift and inspire you, whether they are friends, family, or support groups. A reliable network helps you feel connected and supported, offering valuable perspectives and practical help during difficult times.

1. Set Realistic Goals and Celebrate Achievements: Establishing achievable goals provides direction and motivation. Break larger goals into smaller, manageable steps and celebrate your progress. Recognizing and celebrating your achievements, no matter how small reinforces your sense of accomplishment and strengthens your resilience.

1. Practice Mindfulness and Stress Management: Incorporate mindfulness practices such as meditation, deep breathing exercises, or yoga into your routine. These techniques help you stay grounded and manage stress effectively. Mindfulness encourages you to focus on the present moment, reducing anxiety and enhancing your ability to handle challenges with a calm and balanced perspective.

Seeking professional help, when necessary, ensures you have the resources to continue building and sustaining resilience over time.

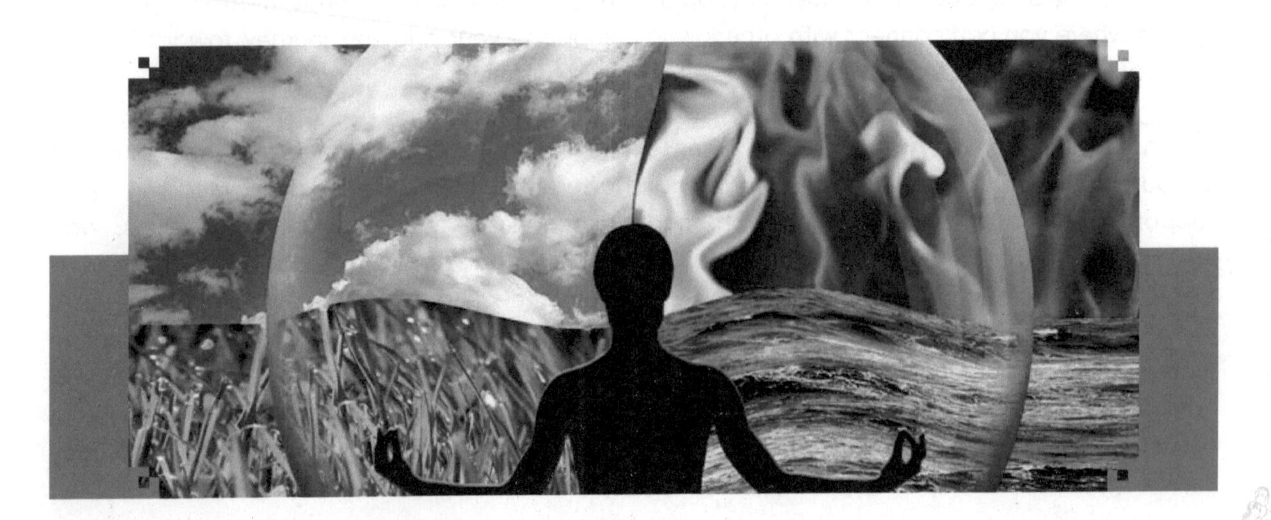

Chapter 9

Building Healthy Relationships

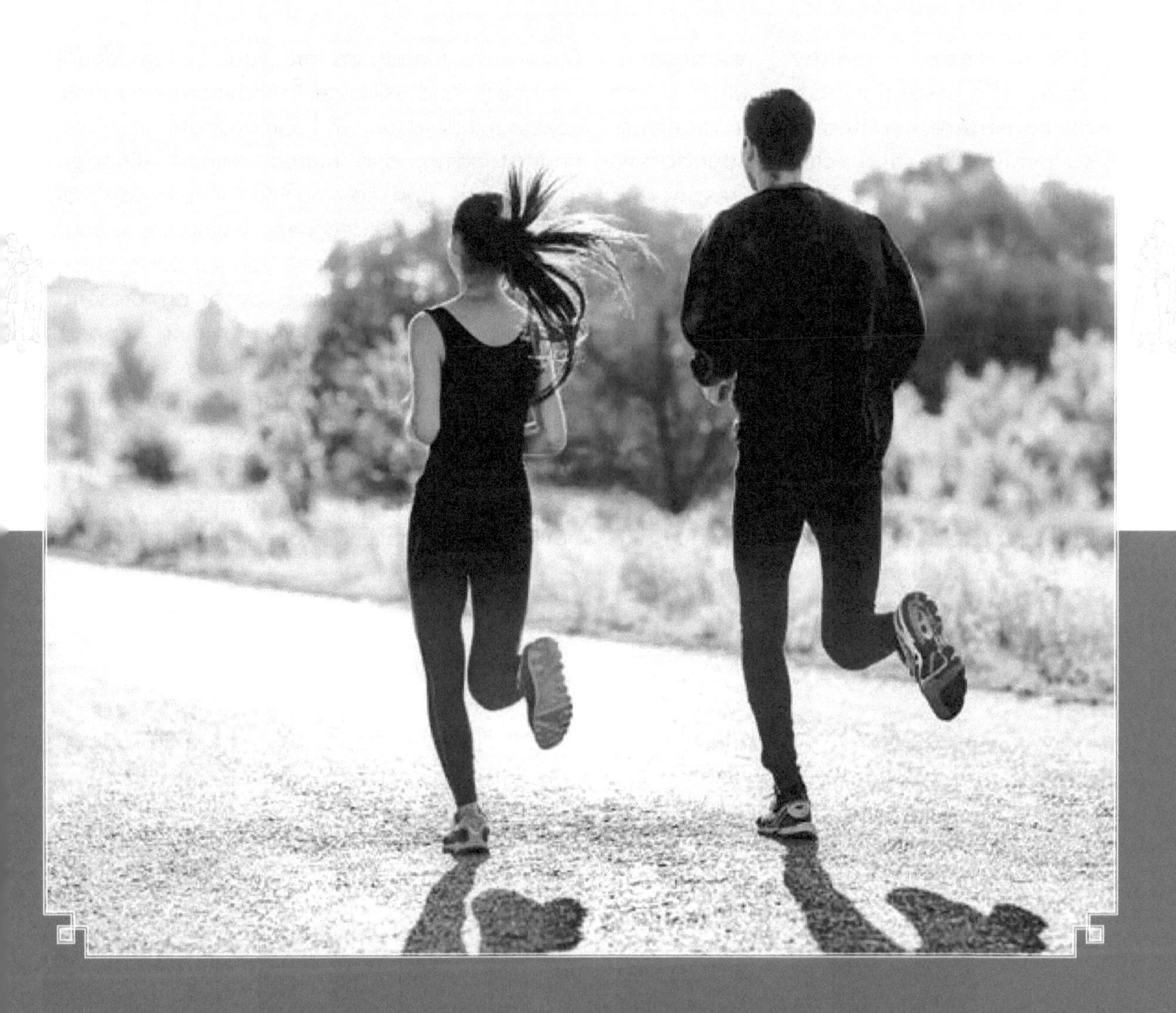

Building healthy relationships is a crucial aspect of healing and personal growth, especially for those who have experienced toxic dynamics in their past. Developing new, positive relationship patterns, enhancing communication, finding supportive friendships, and establishing trust are all critical elements in creating meaningful connections. Here's how to approach each aspect:

Forming New, Healthy Relationship Patterns

To form new, healthy relationship patterns, it's essential first to understand what constitutes a healthy relationship. This involves setting clear boundaries, recognizing your own needs, and respecting those of others. Start by identifying and addressing any old patterns or behaviors that past toxic relationships might have influenced. Engage in self-reflection to understand how these patterns affect your current relationships. Practice being mindful of your interactions, ensuring they are based on mutual respect and understanding. By consciously creating and nurturing these positive dynamics, you build a foundation for healthier relationships.

The Role of Communication in Healthy Relationships

Effective communication is the cornerstone of any healthy relationship. It involves not only expressing your own needs and feelings clearly but also actively listening to others. Open, honest communication fosters understanding and helps prevent misunderstandings and conflicts. Use "I" statements to express your thoughts and feelings, which helps avoid blame and encourages constructive dialogue. Practice active listening by giving your full attention, validating the other person's perspective, and responding thoughtfully. Communication also involves non-verbal cues, such as body language and facial expressions, which can significantly impact how your messages are received.

Finding and Nurturing Supportive Friendships

Supportive friendships are vital for emotional well-being and resilience. To find such friendships, seek out individuals who demonstrate empathy, understanding, and mutual respect. Engage in activities and communities where you will likely meet like-minded people who share your values and interests. Once you establish these connections, nurture them by being present, showing appreciation, and providing support in return. Building and maintaining supportive friendships involves regular communication, shared experiences, and a genuine interest in each other's well-being. These friendships create a network of support that can help you navigate life's challenges and celebrate its joys.

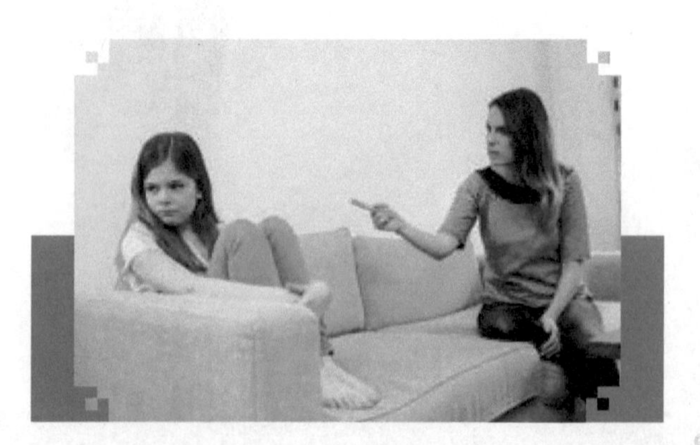

Identifying and Avoiding Toxic Relationships

Identifying and avoiding toxic relationships is crucial for maintaining your emotional health. Patterns of manipulation, control, or emotional abuse characterize poisonous relationships. Look for signs such as constant criticism, lack of respect for boundaries, and a consistent pattern of negative interactions. Trust your instincts—it may be toxic if a relationship consistently leaves you feeling drained or undervalued. Establishing clear boundaries and asserting your needs can help you distance yourself from harmful dynamics. Priorities relationships that contribute positively to your life and align with your values.

Building Trust and Intimacy

Building trust and intimacy requires time, patience, and mutual effort. Trust is established through consistent, reliable behavior and open communication. Be honest and transparent with your feelings and actions to foster a sense of reliability. Intimacy grows from shared experiences, emotional vulnerability, and a deep understanding of each other's needs and desires. Engage in meaningful conversations, express your feelings openly, and create opportunities for connection and shared experiences. Trust and intimacy are nurtured through mutual respect, active listening, and a willingness to work through challenges together.

In summary, building healthy relationships involves forming new, positive patterns, embracing effective communication, and nurturing supportive friendships. Identifying and avoiding toxic relationships is crucial for maintaining emotional health while building trust and intimacy requires honesty, transparency, and shared experiences. By focusing on these aspects, you can create meaningful and fulfilling relationships that contribute positively to your well-being and personal growth.

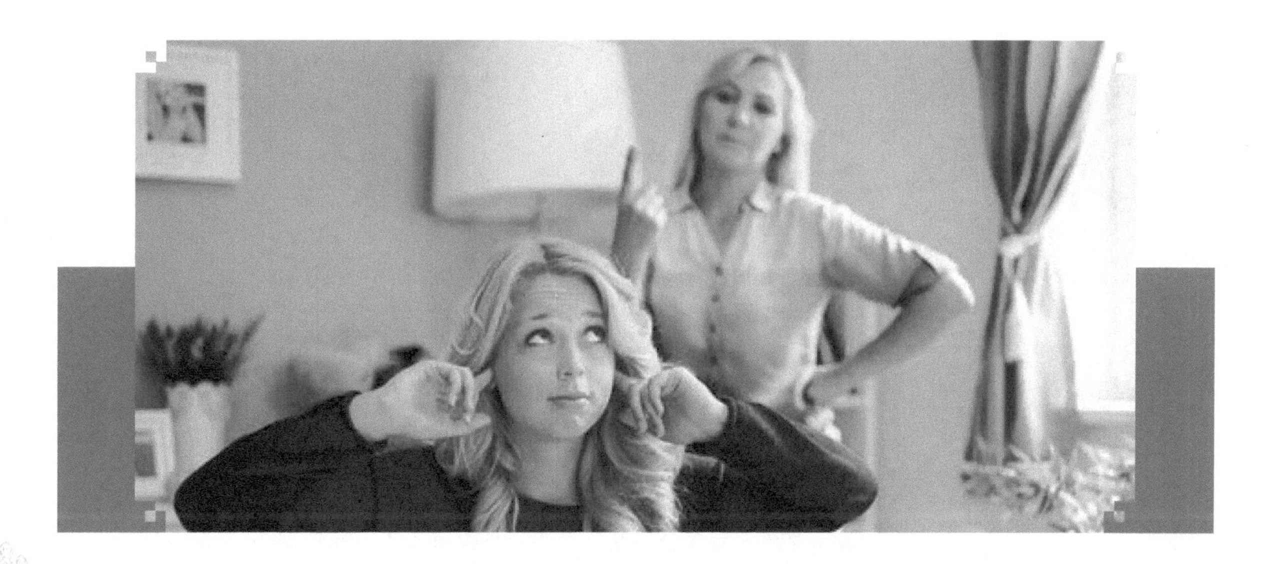

Chapter 10

Moving Forward

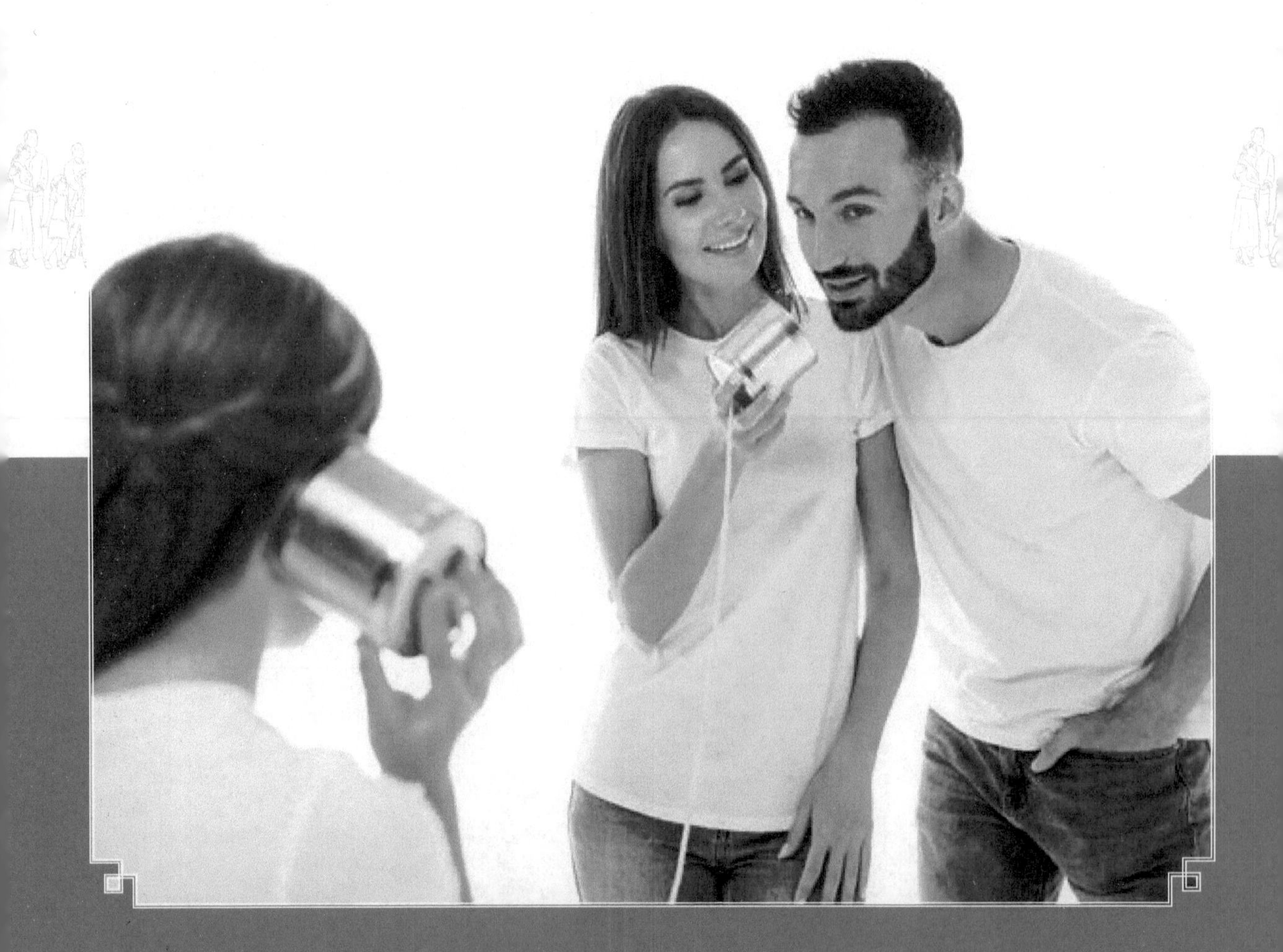

Transitioning from a life impacted by toxic relationships to one of personal growth and fulfilment involves embracing change, setting meaningful goals, and maintaining a positive mindset. Moving forward means actively working towards a future that reflects your values and aspirations while celebrating your journey. Here's how to navigate this process effectively:

Embracing Your New Life

Embracing your new life starts with accepting the changes that come with personal growth and healing. This involves letting go of past hurts and adopting a forward-focused mindset. Embrace the opportunities that arise from your journey, and recognize the strengths and insights you've gained. Acknowledge the positive changes in your life and integrate them into your daily routine. Doing so creates a foundation for a fulfilling and authentic life that aligns with your true self.

Setting Goals for Personal Growth and Fulfillment

Setting goals is a crucial step in moving forward. Start by identifying areas where you wish to grow or achieve fulfilment. These goals should be specific, measurable, attainable, relevant, and time-bound (SMART). Break them down into smaller, manageable steps, and create a plan to achieve them. Setting clear goals provides direction and motivation, whether related to career aspirations, personal development, or relationships. Regularly review and adjust your goals as needed to ensure they continue to reflect your evolving desires and values.

Celebrating Your Progress and Successes

Acknowledging and celebrating your progress is vital for maintaining motivation and reinforcing positive changes. Take time to reflect on your achievements, no matter how small they may seem. Celebrate milestones by rewarding yourself or sharing your successes with loved ones. Recognizing your progress boosts your confidence and reinforces your commitment to personal growth. Keep a journal or create a visual representation of your achievements to remind yourself how far you've come.

Developing a Positive Mindset

A positive mindset is essential for navigating challenges and sustaining personal growth. Focus on cultivating an optimistic outlook by practicing gratitude, reframing negative thoughts, and celebrating your strengths. Surround yourself with positive influences and engage in activities that uplift and inspire you. A positive mindset helps you approach obstacles with resilience and fosters a greater sense of fulfilment and happiness.

Long-term Strategies for Maintaining Emotional Health

Maintaining emotional health over the long term requires ongoing effort and self-care. Develop and adhere to self-care routines that support your physical, emotional, and mental well-being. This includes regular exercise, healthy eating, mindfulness practices, and hobbies. Additionally, continue building and nurturing supportive relationships that provide encouragement and understanding. Seek professional support when needed, and stay proactive in addressing emerging challenges. Integrating these strategies into your life creates a sustainable framework for ongoing emotional health and resilience.

Chapter 11

Resources for Further Support

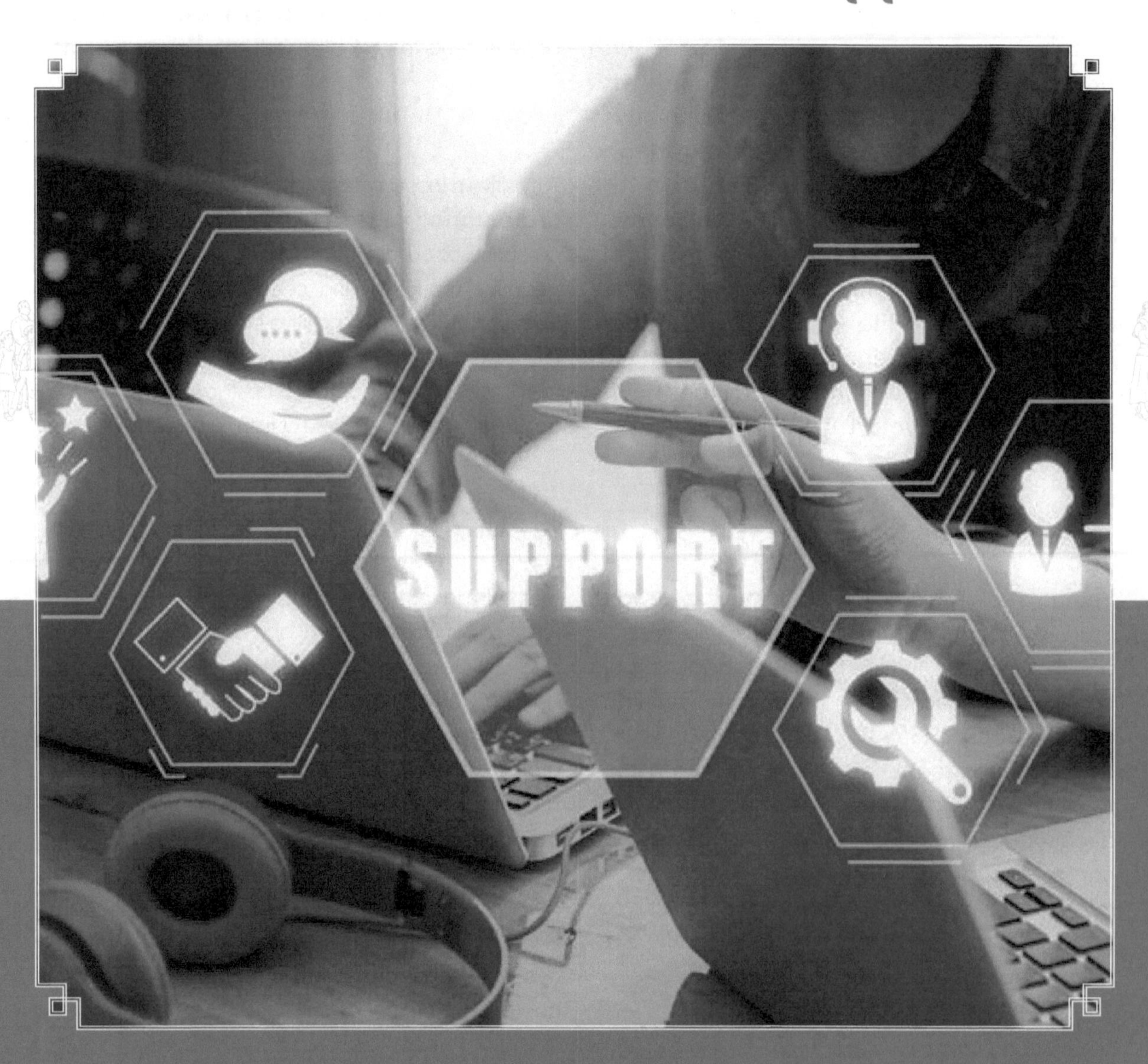

Navigating the journey of healing and personal growth is a multifaceted process that can benefit from additional resources and support. The following resources provide valuable tools and connections to help you continue toward emotional well-being and fulfilment.

Recommended Books

Books can offer insight, strategies, and comfort as you face challenges. Here are some recommended reads that cover various aspects of personal growth, healing from toxic relationships, and building emotional resilience:

"The Body Keeps the Score" by Bessel van der Kolk, M.D. – Explores how trauma affects the body and mind and offers insights into healing.

"Radical Acceptance" by Tara Brach – Provides tools for embracing your life and accepting yourself with compassion.

"Adult Children of Emotionally Immature Parents" by Lindsay C. Gibson, PsyD – Offers guidance on understanding and dealing with the impact of emotionally immature parents.

"The Gifts of Imperfection" by Brené Brown – Focuses on embracing vulnerability and cultivating a wholehearted life.

"The Four Agreements" by Don Miguel Ruiz – Discusses practical principles for personal freedom and a fulfilling life.

Online Support Groups

Connecting with others who share similar experiences can provide valuable support and encouragement. Online support groups offer a space to share, seek advice, and find solidarity. Consider joining:

Reddit Communities (e.g., r/ADHD, r/Emotional Intelligence) – These forums offer discussions on various topics related to emotional health and personal growth.

Daily Strength (dailystrength.org) – Provides support groups and resources for various mental health and personal development issues.

Mental Health America Support Groups (mhanational.org) – Offers online communities to discuss mental health challenges and find support.

Support Groups Central (supportgroupscentral.com) – Connects you with online groups for emotional and psychological support.

Online Resources and Communities

The internet offers many resources for learning and connecting with others on your healing journey. Explore these websites for valuable information and community support:

Psychology Today (psychologytoday.com) – Features articles, therapist directories, and resources on mental health topics.

Midbudget (mindbodygreen.com) – Provides articles and advice on holistic health and wellness.

NAMI (National Alliance on Mental Illness) (nami.org) – Offers resources and support for various mental health conditions, including links to local support groups.

The Center for Self-Compassion (centerforselfcompassion.org) – Provides resources and tools for cultivating self-compassion.

Apps and Tools for Emotional Health

Technology can support your emotional well-being through various apps and tools to promote mental health and personal growth. Consider trying:

Headspace – A meditation app offering guided mindfulness and relaxation exercises.

Calm – Provides meditation, sleep stories, and relaxation techniques to manage stress and anxiety.

Mood fit – Tracks your mood, provides mental health resources, and helps you develop coping strategies.

Reflect – A journaling app that encourages self-reflection and helps track your emotional state.

7 Cups – Connects you with trained listeners for emotional support and offers self-help resources.

Building Your Support Network

Creating a strong support network is a cornerstone of maintaining emotional health and navigating the complexities of personal growth. Such a network provides a safety net during challenging times and enriches your life with connection, understanding, and encouragement. Here's a deeper look at how to build and nurture this essential support system:

REACH OUT TO FRIENDS AND FAMILY

Your close relationships are vital sources of support. Engage with those who offer genuine understanding and empathy. Open up about your experiences, fears, and aspirations. Sharing your journey with loved ones can be both cathartic and affirming. When you ask for help, you allow others to support you meaningfully, strengthening your bond and fostering a sense of mutual care. Remember, seeking support is not a sign of weakness; it's a brave step towards healing and growth.

JOIN LOCAL OR ONLINE GROUPS

Connecting with people with similar interests or challenges can provide a sense of belonging and camaraderie. Look for local meetups, community events, or online forums that resonate with your passions and experiences. Engaging in these groups can offer both practical advice and emotional comfort. Through these interactions, you find validation, encouragement, and a sense of community that can uplift your spirit and broaden your perspectives.

SEEK PROFESSIONAL GUIDANCE

Therapists and counsellors offer specialized support tailored to your needs. They provide a safe space to explore your thoughts and feelings, and their guidance can help you develop effective coping strategies. Professional support is critical to your healing journey, offering insights and tools that empower you to navigate your challenges with confidence and resilience. Don't hesitate to reach out for this kind of support—it's an investment in your well-being and future.

VOLUNTEER OR GET INVOLVED

Volunteering and getting involved in causes you care about can be incredibly fulfilling. It allows you to connect with like-minded individuals who share your values and passions. This engagement enriches your life with purpose and helps build a supportive community around you. By contributing to meaningful causes, you positively impact others and find a more profound sense of connection and belonging.

In summary, nurturing a strong support network is crucial for sustaining your emotional well-being and continuing your journey of personal growth. Leveraging various resources, including recommended books, online support groups, and professional guidance, enhances your path towards healing. You build a resilient network that provides ongoing encouragement and strength by contacting friends and family, participating in local or online groups, seeking professional support, and engaging in volunteer work. This support system is not just about finding help; it's about fostering relationships and connections that sustain you through the highs and lows of life, reinforcing your sense of purpose and belonging.

Conclusion

One final thing to do before turning the last page of this book is to meditate deeply on the experience you have just been offered. The difficulties of recovering from the experiences and relational trauma that result from toxic relationships, as well as the process of regaining one's emotional sovereignty, must not be underestimated. It is an act of courage and defiance that comes with admission of personal sadness and institutional fortitude. Although it can be difficult, it is an essential transformational process that has the potential to change the person for the better.

All these chapters in this book have helped you dive deep into the complexity of guilt and shame, learn about self-compassion and find effective ways of developing healthy relationships. But each is the step to healing, as each provides you with the understanding of yourself and your feelings and the tools to face the world. This road to healing is very individual; people must search inside themselves, try, and be strong enough to heal themselves.

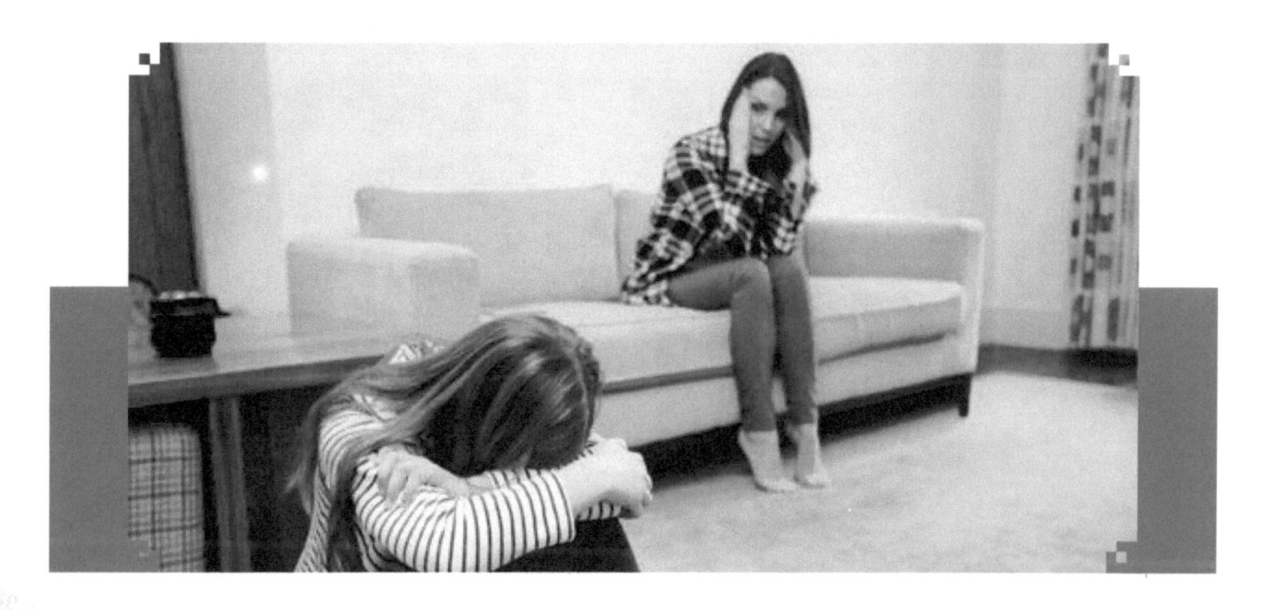

Getting over the heartbreak is not easy, and it is a proven fact that the process is usually winding. It snakes through laps of victory and phases of adversity of its climax and trough. This journey has made you face your dark side, change your ways of thinking and perceiving reality, and, ultimately, embrace yourself for the better self you are becoming. Ever since you have displayed such a marked ability to change and develop. I appreciate your efforts in dealing with your pain, as well as your desire to take a closer look at your feelings and change unhealthy patterns.

Another one of the most prominent elements driving your process has been the concept of self-care. Understanding one's human nature, accepting oneself, being kind to oneself, and forgiving one's mistakes have been enlightening and liberating. It is not a strategy that stops as soon as depressive thoughts come to an end; it outlines an entirely different approach to how a person is treated. This shift has helped you to grow and recover from the past to a level that could stand afresh with hope and strength. So, by accepting self-compassion, you have achieved the framework for a lifetime of positive mental and emotional health.

Reestablishing one's independent self has also posted significant importance in healing; this includes forming new and healthy relationships. In establishing the limits, sharing your needs, and creating positive interactions, you have built the foundation of the relationships encompassing who you are. These relationships are not just avenues of comfort but part and parcel of one's well-being and human development. They give approval and support and make your life much more worthwhile in ways you never thought of. This ability to start and maintain these relations is a true sign of how strong or accurate you have grown.

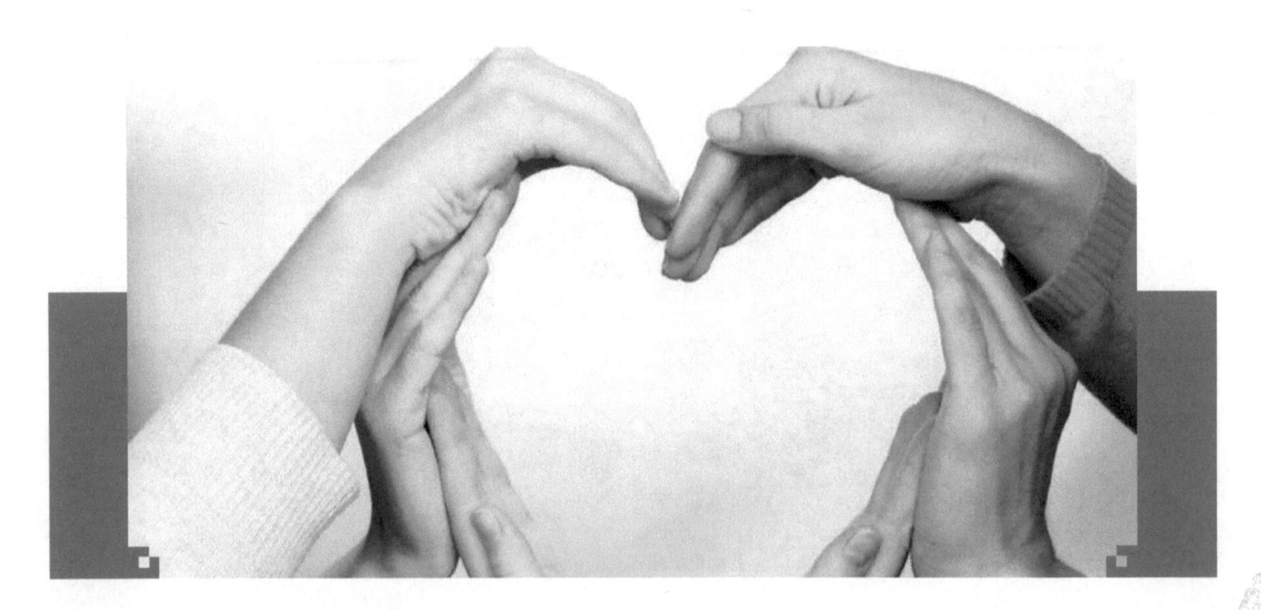

Living our new lives also entails accepting the changes we have made and the people we have transformed into. The gap refers to admitting the capability and fortitude that one has built and enabling oneself to be fully ready to take on the future. This new chapter of your life is your story of braving the uncertainty and paving the way to the life you envision for yourself. It is an opportunity to celebrate who a person is now and the evolution that leads to that stage in life.

Recognition of the kind is the critical component of this process. All the actions you are making now towards healing, all that has been bothering you, which you have tackled head and tackled, and every achievement you have ever made is a victory. Such celebrations are not just fun; they are ways of acknowledging your victories; woman, you are strong. They encourage you to reach out for more and help you recall what you can do. Job well done. My only regret is that I am not a partaker of those celebrations. They are a clear testimony and confirmation of your hard work and dedication to embracing the fruits of a purposeful and fulfilling life.

Therefore, it is essential to note that preserving one's emotional well-being is a complicated process that entails consistent dedication. The Advanced Level strategies and tools you have learned in this book will go a long way in further development. It is essential to support one's physical and mental health and care for people with whom one maintains close contact and stays active when facing any issues. It might not be a one-time trip, and each day could be a new day that brings new experiences and opportunities to make a new change. Remember that a form of emotional health is not a destination but a journey that we are on and needs consistent effort.

Merry Christmas. As you look to the future, do not allow anybody to determine the course of your life. You have been prepared well for life's challenges in every way, knowledgeably, physically, and spiritually, enabling you to conquer life in a dignified manner. Accept future chances that will come your way as you believe you can build a wonderful, loving life. This must be viewed as your story of bravery, change and optimism. It portrays how you can reclaim your life after something wrong and build a new life for yourself and your loved ones.

Onward as you go, I hope you discover meaning in the process, the power of a struggle and the comfort in knowing that all people deserve a life filled with love and relationships. It only remains for me to say thank you for giving this book a place in your life. The brighter days are ahead of you, and only your improvement and inner healing can prove there is so much more in you than you know. Welcome the next phase of your life with a happy attitude and optimism, as the next phase of life is full of more opportunities to learn, discover and be satisfied. Your ability to get back up has helped you come this far and will keep bringing you to where you wish to be as a fulfilled person.

Jacqueline D. Austin

Made in United States
Troutdale, OR
01/04/2025